Primary Health Care Sciences

Primary Health Care Sciences

Edited by

Jane Sims PhD MSc BSc(Hons)

Department of General Practice and Primary Care
St George's Hospital Medical School, London

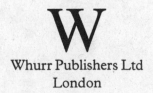

Whurr Publishers Ltd
London

© 1999 Whurr Publishers
First published 1999 by
Whurr Publishers Ltd
19b Compton Terrace, London N1 2UN, England

British Library Cataloguing in Publication Data
A catalogue record for this book is available from the British
Library.

ISBN: 1 86156 103 2

Contents

Contributors

Elizabeth ARMSTRONG RGN, RHV, is at the National Depression Care Training Centre, Nene University College, Northampton. She is also Mental Health Training Officer for the National Primary Care Facilitation Programme and Honorary Tutor in Psychiatric Nursing at the Institute of Psychiatry, London.

Christine BOND PhD, is Acting Chief Administrative Pharmaceutical Officer and Lecturer in the Department of General Practice, University of Aberdeen.

Naomi FULOP PhD, is Senior Lecturer in the Health Services Research Unit, Department of Public Health and Policy, at the London School of Hygiene and Tropical Medicine.

Pat GORDON is Director of Primary Care at the King's Fund, London.

Geoff MEADS MA (Oxon), MSc, is Visiting Professor of Health Services Development at City University, London.

Elizabeth MITCHELL BA, is a Research Fellow in the Department of General Practice, University of Glasgow.

Pauline PEARSON PhD, RHV, is Senior Lecturer in Primary Care Nursing in the Department of Primary Health Care at the University of Newcastle upon Tyne.

Fiona ROSS PhD, RGN, DN, is Professor of Primary Care Nursing in the Faculty of Healthcare Sciences at St George's Hospital Medical School, London.

Jane SIMS PhD, is Lecturer in Primary Health Care Sciences in the Department of General Practice and Primary Care at St George's Hospital Medical School, London.

Frank SULLIVAN PhD, FRCP, FRCGP, is Professor of Research and Development in General Practice and Primary Care at the Tayside Centre for General Practice, University of Dundee.

André TYLEE MBBS, MRCPsych, FRCGP, is Director of the RCGP Mental Health Education Unit at the Institute of Psychiatry, University of London.

Patricia WILKIE MA, PhD, is Chairman of the Patients Liaison Group at the Royal College of General Practitioners and an advisor to the patients group at the Royal College of Radiologists, where she is also a Council member.

Acknowledgements

I would like to thank the contributors for all their hard work in helping this book come to fruition. A number of people have provided support and advice during the development of this book. I am particularly grateful for the comments of Dr Anthony Mathie, Dr Oliver Samuels and Andrew Singleton.

The evaluation of the hospital-at-home schemes in West London described in Chapter 7 was funded by North Thames R&D Organisational and Management Group. The author would like to acknowledge the help of colleagues on the study: Sonja Hood, Sharon Parsons, Martin Hensher and Helen Hunter. The author would also like to thank Aileen Clarke, Judy Green, Rebecca Rosen and Sasha Shepperd for their help and advice.

Preface

The past decade has seen a number of changes in the provision of primary health care, triggered to some degree by the ideological concept of a primary care-led NHS. The players and the tasks within primary care have been realigned to meet the challenge of providing more health care within this arena. Whilst the GP remains a key player in primary health care delivery, there has been a move towards increased collaboration across professional boundaries and the integration of health professionals' roles to promote more seamless care. The systems of care have also undergone development to incorporate new means of organizing care both within primary care and across the primary—secondary care interface. Within the organizational structure, tools such as guidelines have been introduced to assist in giving good-quality, cost-effective care.

This changing landscape has called for radical moves in the areas of education, audit and research. Members of the primary health care team need to be adequately supported if they are to respond to the emerging doctrines and political imperatives. Thorough needs assessment, audit and evaluation should accompany any major modification to the conditions under which health care is conducted. There have been a variety of ventures to promote evidence-based practice: these are set to continue.

So, what are primary health care sciences? Science itself has many definitions, and the term has evoked much controversy. Here the phrase broadly encompasses the discovery, creation, accumulation and refinement of knowledge pertinent to primary health care. This book aims to add to primary care epistemology, that is, the study of such knowledge, although it does so from a practical rather than a philosophical basis.

The study of primary health care encompasses a broad array of paradigms, from the behavioural and social sciences, through to the clinical sciences. It embraces philosophies and principles from the disciplines of anthropology, sociology, psychology, ethics, health economics, business management and education. The professionals working in primary care comprise specialists from all of these fields. Any one individual health professional's perspective will be influenced by the dominant discipline that has shaped his or her education. One aim of this book is to encourage readers to think beyond their familiar paradigms, since there are various ways of understanding problems, both within and between disciplines.

Theories are developed to explain the relationships of observable phenomena and to predict future events from present knowledge. A theory is a system of rules, procedures and assumptions used to explain relations between phenomena. Simply speaking, theories are statements about how the world 'works'. Whilst theories have undoubtedly driven primary health care developments, they have not, generally speaking, done so explicitly. For example, the important contribution of theories from the humanities and social and organizational sciences needs to be unveiled. The prevailing opacity poses difficulties for the observer who wishes to understand what is guiding primary health care. Perhaps more transparent are some of the models that have aided the application of theory. A model is a means of representing theory to allow it to be studied, understood and tested. For example, the dominant paradigm for the doctor is based upon the medical model.

At a further level of understanding, we have concepts. A concept is an abstract idea that categorizes data and enables generalization from particulars. Core concepts in primary care include communication and social networks, health beliefs and empowerment, health technology and quality development, economics and priority-setting. Primary health care professionals have a variety of frameworks for codifying concepts, experiences and the information that organizes how they perceive, learn and remember.

The content of this book serves to illustrate the variety of perspectives in primary health care. A number of the chapters explicitly mention theories, models and concepts. Readers will see that much of the impetus for primary health care change has been political and legislative, rather than theory driven. It would therefore be artificial to conduct a *post hoc* 'pigeon-holing' of emerging concepts. Nevertheless, the reader may wish to reflect upon and research further the important influences.

A number of key experts and researchers in the field of primary health care have contributed to this book. Drawing on their collective knowledge, the chapters address a variety of important issues, ranging from interprofessional working to new technology. The book provides a useful overview of the recent transformations in primary health care. It brings together in one text a discussion of the important changes, with a commentary from those who have been closely involved in monitoring them. It will be helpful to all professionals working in primary health care and to all those interested in the impact of primary care on other areas of the National Health Service. The emphasis is upon the UK scene, although some of the alterations noted are also taking place elsewhere.

There are a number of themes within this book. The first two chapters review the historical background and the organizational changes occurring over the past two decades. The following four chapters deal more closely with professional and service issues arising from the various policy changes. The next three chapters discuss a number of novel approaches to promote efficient care giving and describe how the patient is increasingly an active participant rather than a passive recipient of such innovations. The final chapter takes up an issue arising from earlier chapters and considers the implications of a changing health service upon the educational needs of primary health care professionals, using GP education as an exemplar.

Chapter 1 gives the historical perspective, outlining the various political and legislative stimuli underpinning the alterations in primary health care practice. It notes how social and community services increasingly support the general practice infrastructure. It focuses on the impact of fundholding, commissioning and the 1990 GP contract, and reflects upon barriers to implementing policy.

Chapter 2 discusses the modified role of the GP in the light of policy-driven deregulation and the devolution of responsibility for service provision. The importance of nationwide equity of quality of care is emphasized. The history of GP fundholding is summarized, and the development of commissioning, which will form the basis of the emerging primary care groups, is discussed. The remoulding of NHS primary care based upon organizational psychology and social theory is noted.

Chapter 3 investigates how policy changes have modified the role of the nurse in the primary health care arena and discusses how the profession is reshaping both its training and practice. The evolution of care assessment and management protocols to enhance continuity of care using a team approach is highlighted.

Chapter 4 explores the increasing potential for involvement in primary health care of the professions allied to medicine. Aspects of skill mix and interprofessional collaboration via teamwork are considered. The theoretical basis of interprofessional working is discussed.

Chapter 5 notes the shift in emphasis being proffered by the Royal Pharmaceutical Society of Great Britain for the pharmacist's role in primary care. Increasing use of the community pharmacist in health promotion and closer ties with other members of the primary health care team are discussed. Inter- and intraprofessional barriers to change are discussed.

Chapter 6 focuses on mental health, an area that is increasingly being managed within primary care. The implications of this are considered and innovative systems of care delivery discussed.

In Chapter 7, aspects of care across the primary—secondary care interface are illustrated by a discussion of hospital-at-home services. The rationale for and the development and monitoring of such systems of care are outlined.

Chapter 8 draws together details of a number of innovations in new technology designed to facilitate good practice in primary care. These include patient testing, decision support systems and interactive educational packages.

Chapter 9 gives the patient perspective on primary health care transformations. The role of the patient as a consumer and patients' impact via participation in health care are reviewed.

Chapter 10 reflects on the educational needs of health professionals working in the 'new' NHS. GP training is used as an example. An overview of historical, current and emerging trends in medical education is provided.

This book brings together representatives from various key professions to give their unique perspectives on the current trends in primary health care in a discourse which, it is hoped, will benefit those from allied professions. This book will be useful for all students at undergraduate and post-graduate level who wish to improve their understanding of contemporary issues in primary health care. It should be particularly helpful to those taking part in the growing number of interprofessional educational programmes. It is intended to support the underlying philosophy of these courses: that of promoting better health care via interprofessional collaboration and the engendering of a greater understanding of the roles of other health professionals.

Editorial note

This book was written during 1996/1997, when the NHS White Papers were a first a glint in the Health Secretary's eye and then published for the mental digestion of all. Where appropriate, the contributors have speculated upon the impact of the contents for primary care. It will be appreciated that the NHS is a dynamic setting. During 1998 there have been many debates, focusing on such issues as clinical governance, self-regulation and the role of the Commission for Health Improvement, to be established as an independent statutory body in 1999/2000. Until these changes get underway, it will not be possible to evaluate whether – and if so, how – the global policy objective of 'quality in the NHS' has been met. It is hoped that future editions of this book will offer objective commentary upon the emerging changes particularly in relation to primary care groups. There will also be scope for reflection upon the allied public health proposals, outlined in the Green Paper *Our Healthier Nation*.

The book refers to individuals in general in the masculine throughout. This has been done for ease of reading and does not denote any gender bias.

Chapter 1
Primary care in context

Pat Gordon

Introduction

Primary care services form the infrastructure of most health care systems. What varies is the strength of that infrastructure. In a study of 11 Western industrialized nations, Barbara Starfield shows that a strong primary care system is not only linked to better health outcomes for the population, but also associated with lower costs (Starfield, 1995). She argues that a strong primary care service providing the first level of care in a health system is more effective, more efficient and more equitable than a system oriented towards direct access to specialists.

In the UK, primary care services are generally seen as the foundation for the appropriate use of the specialist/hospital sector and therefore for the effective management of its costs. In its planning guidance to the end of 20th century, the National Health Service Executive (NHSE) lists its first priority as 'a primary care-led NHS where decisions about health care are taken as close to patients as possible' (National Health Service Executive, 1995). However, there is considerable confusion about what the phrase 'a primary care-led NHS' means and how it might be implemented. This is at least in part because of the great variation in the quality and structure of general practices and community health services across the country. General practice and community health services Trusts, along with health authorities, are generally assumed to be the means through which this policy will be delivered. Most health authority managers, however, have made their careers in the hospital sector, so it is not surprising that there is uncertainty, doubt, curiosity and a great deal of speculation about the future shape of a primary care-led NHS. The dramatic changes to the NHS in the 1990s have started a trend that looks set

1

to continue well into the next century, the only certainty being that there will be no single blueprint. The phrases may change, but the drive for a strong primary care infrastructure will not recede because it is seen internationally as the means, for the foreseeable future, of containing costs and improving health (Starfield, 1994).

Definitions are sometimes helpful, and here it seems worth making the distinction between the terms 'primary care' and 'primary health care'. Primary care is used to describe the patient's first point of contact with the health care services. This contrasts with secondary care, which is the layer of services, often but not always hospital-based, to which patients may be referred from primary care. In the UK, the main primary care provider organizations are general practice, community health services Trusts, pharmacists, opticians, dentists and hospital accident and emergency departments. The term 'primary care' is often equated simply with general practice, or even more simply with GPs.

Primary health care is a much broader concept, as described in the 1978 World Health Organisation conference at Alma Ata (World Health Organisation, 1978). It rests on three principles of participation, intersectoral collaboration and equity. It is an approach that emphasizes the promotion of health through partnership and is seen as the means of attaining a level of health that would allow everyone to lead a socially and economically viable life.

This chapter discusses the characteristics of primary care and what patients value about it. It goes on to describe the main providers of primary care in the UK – general practice and the community health services – and their connections into the social care and hospital care networks. It offers an historical perspective on how services developed in the UK as a guide to understanding how they might change to meet the NHS policy priority. The reforms of the 1990s are put into the context of the pressures for change in health care systems in all industrialized societies in recent years. The chapter ends with a discussion of the 1996 White Papers and the possible deregulation of primary care in the NHS.

The vast majority of health services in the UK are provided 'in the community'. More than that, when people are ill or distressed, most care is provided by family and friends. In a paper on shifting the balance 'from acute to community health care', Boufford (1994) describes the classic study analysing the sickness behaviour of 1000 adults over 16 years of age in 1 month using the Survey of Sickness in England and Wales and the US National Health Survey. Of the thousand, 750 people experienced some health complaint, 250 of those sought medical attention, 9 of those were admitted to a community hospital, 5 were referred to another physician and 1 was admitted to a teaching hospital (White et al, 1961). On this basis, fewer than 4% of people who enter the formal health care system need a hospital. Boufford refers to a similar review with a similar pattern 20 years later, in 1983, and uses 1990s relative activity figures for the NHS to show some 216 million consultations with GPs and 17 million contacts with community health and other paramedical professionals, compared with 7.7 million in-patient episodes, 1.6 million day cases and 20 million new out-patient and accident and emergency attendances in 1991–92. On this evidence, most people's experience of the NHS takes place in what we can call the primary care system. Understanding its main characteristics and what patients value about it may help to put some of the policy changes of the past few years into context.

Primary care offers *first contact care* and is the patient's first point of entry to the health system. It takes place in many different places, large and small, private homes and public clinics, often far from the offices and institutions where many of us work. Because it takes place 'out there', it is not as visible as hospital care, nor is it the province of one group of professionals. It can be described as a network of community-based health services that covers the prevention of ill-health, the treatment of acute and chronic illness, the promotion of health, rehabilitation, support at home for frail people, the management of long-term ill-health, and terminal care. At its best, this network works with and through general practice to deliver services and to access secondary care, and is in turn linked to an even wider social care network. Primary care is complex, organic, small and local. It is multi-professional, multi-agency, multi-shaped and multi-sized. As long as services reach an agreed standard, diversity in primary care is a welcome and appropriate characteristic in local organizations striving to meet local needs.

Coulter (1996) describes an ideal model of primary care in which:

> primary care teams provide continuous care and preventive services for defined populations, referring on to specialist services only where necessary. The emphasis is on co-ordination and continuity of services, which respect individuals' autonomy while catering for the full range of basic health needs for local populations. At its best, a strong primary care system should be able to deliver cost-effective health care distributed equitably according to need.

Doctors, nurses and many of the professions supplementary to medicine who deliver primary care services are trained in the 'biomedical approach', which includes technical competence, a knowledge base and action in the perceived best interests of the individual patient. As the knowledge and skills base of biomedical science has grown during the 20th century, so has the need for specialists. In general, patients can access a range of medical specialists in one of two ways. The first is directly, as happens in the USA, by deciding which speciality is appropriate and relying on the specialist to manage the illness or refer to another specialist. The other route, more common in the UK, is to consult a generalist who is able to manage common problems and knows when it is appropriate to refer and to which specialist. One of the strengths of this latter approach is that it acknowledges that many patients bring problems from more than one speciality and that much of the illness and distress that patients feel is not amenable to biomedical intervention (Pratt, 1995).

General practice offers primary care delivered by clinical generalists who, in addition to a biomedical approach, can offer continuing and personal care for patients. This is often described as 'biographical care' and allows episodes of illness to be understood in the context of people's daily lives. Pratt has described a set of values of the clinical generalist that include accepting any problem brought by the patient that might be amenable to biomedical intervention, availability, mutual trust, continuity of care, responsibility for the co-ordination of care of the individual patient, and the ability to tolerate uncertainty (Pratt, 1995). This biographical approach is often described as being patient centred.

Another characteristic of general practice is to offer accessible care. This means not only geographical nearness, but also availability, language, culture and concern for old as well as new health problems. Part of the accessibility is to do with general practices being small, local organizations whose scale is important in maintaining the non-institutional, personal care that many patients value.

The characteristic of comprehensive care is not defined by sickness, age, race or gender. It includes disease prevention, health promotion, the treatment of acute and chronic illness and rehabilitation. The availability of services 24 hours a day is part of this comprehensiveness and is one way of reducing self-referral to other services. Comprehensive care involves teamwork, in which a growing number of professionals share aspects of patient care.

Since patients frequently present with distress and 'messy' problems that do not lend themselves to neat or simple solutions, another attribute of good general practice is co-ordinated care. Heath (1993) has described the GP as the 'guardian of the interface between illness and disease'. The practitioner will work with the patient to enable him to make sense of the problem, and will sometimes act as information-giver or advocate. Co-ordinated care also includes referral for specialist care.

The community health services bring another set of characteristics to primary care. They are provided by larger organizations that cater for larger populations than general practice. The range of professional staff is wide and encompasses a vast array of skills and both specialist and generalist knowledge, for example:

- nurses, who include district nurses, health visitors, community midwives, community psychiatric nurses, MacMillan and Marie Curie nurses, family planning nurses, stoma care nurses, continence advisors and paediatric, diabetic and school nurses;
- professions allied to medicine, who include occupational therapists, chiropodists, physiotherapists, dietitians, speech therapists, psychologists, audiologists, community pharmacists and health promotion staff;
- doctors, who include paediatricians, geriatricians and psychiatrists;
- community dentists.

These staff offer support for general practice, which in small practices can mean employing the district nurse and health visitor, and in large practices can mean service-level agreements for the community psychiatric nurse or midwife. They offer services for people with continuing illness and disability, which often requires skilful networking and liaising with voluntary and local authority agencies. Such staff provide services that support people discharged from hospital, this increasingly taking the form of a vigorous home care programme based on high-quality nursing care. They offer services for people who are well, for example family planning, HIV counselling and school health. There are also community-based specialists such as clinical psychologists and consultant paediatricians. They allow a choice for people without a GP or for those for whom family-based practice may be inappropriate, for example homeless people or young adults seeking advice on sexual health. They offer economies of scale – not every practice wants to employ a physiotherapist, for example, but the patients on every practice list want access to one when needed. Similarly, the appliances and equipment that can enable people to continue living independently in their own homes can only be provided efficiently for a large population. Also, economies of scale allow in-service training and study leave, which may extend to include practice nurses.

General practice and the community health services together form the building blocks of the primary care system in the UK. Between them, they have the potential to deliver the NHS agenda of earlier, safer discharge from hospital, more frail people being supported in their homes, better co-ordinated community care, and a more efficient and effective use of hospital resources (Haggard, 1990). However, the structure and the quality of both general practice and community Trusts varies considerably across the country.

In order to put current events into context and understand how primary care is changing, the next few pages offer a brief historical perspective, based on Gordon and Plamping (1996), on how services have developed in the UK.

An historical perspective of the development of general practice

The roots of general practice are distinct from those of both physicians and surgeons, and can be traced back to the apothecaries of the 19th century, and earlier, who diagnosed conditions and recommended treatments as well as preparing and dispensing medically prescribed therapies. In order to protect the public from 'quackery' in the rapidly changing world of Victorian Britain, the 1858 Medical Requisition Act was passed to help guarantee basic standards of medical qualification and practice. It also helped to fuse three previously conflicting groups into one medical profession, and 'thereafter demarcation disputes between general practitioners and the more specialised physicians and surgeons were metamorphosed into medical etiquette' (Taylor, 1991).

In the early days of the NHS, the emphasis was on access to health care for all (Titmuss, 1963). Two of the fundamental principles of the NHS were:

1. to divorce health care from personal means (in other words to make access to medical services free, in the belief that this would result in preventive action and therefore improved health for the nation);
2. to ensure that medical services were available to everyone.

Access for all meant a new right to be included on a GP's list. For many people, this represented little more than an extension of 'the panel', the pre-NHS list system to which many families contributed, although, importantly, it was an unstigmatized extension. Within a short space of time, it was possible to register almost the whole population with GPs. The really big change, however, was that the NHS brought access to specialist care in hospitals. This equality was most notable in London 'where an East-Ender could receive care from the same specialist who cared for the King and Queen: a fact not unrelated to today's Londoners' attachment to their specialist centres' (Plamping, 1995a).

An agreement reached between the government and the British Medical Association (BMA) left GPs as independent practitioners who continued on their pre-NHS path separated from the mainstream of NHS policy and finance, which, in turn, paid little attention to the place of primary care in the health system. Most hospital managers probably know little about the first Charter in the NHS, the Doctors Charter of 1966, but without understanding its significance and legacy, it is difficult to understand how our system of general practice has evolved.

During the 1950s and 60s, an extraordinary movement developed within general practice. A remarkable cohort of GP leaders developed a theoretical basis for family medicine and a vision of how the role of a clinical generalist might develop within a national health service (Balint, 1957; Royal College of General Practitioners, 1972). They created a Royal College of General Practitioners (RCGP) and a professional culture of audit and vocational training far ahead of the hospital sector. They challenged the notion of the GP as 'the poor relation' of the hospital specialist. Most remarkably, they 'kept the faith' when most health care systems were turning away from the generalist to an increasing reliance on specialists. It is this gift to the current system which allows us to even contemplate a primary care-led future. Other countries that lost their generalists, most notably the USA, face a 20-year development cycle to rebuild an adequate supply (Moore, 1992).

By the mid-1960s, there was a growing awareness within the health service of the importance of the gate-keeping role of the GPs, and this combined with their professional leadership to produce the Charter for general practice. This was a recognition of the need for public spending on general practice buildings, and for access to revenue for staff and equipment, and it marked a significant shift in policy. General practice underwent a renaissance. The best undergraduates began to choose it as a career option. Departments of general practice sprang up in medical schools and further strengthened the theoretical and research base of the profession. In many parts of the country over the next two decades, the range and quality of services blossomed. The new mechanisms were used to create models of care that are recognized as probably the best in the world.

However, it has to be remembered that this was a system built on professional development, which insisted that independent practitioner status was necessary to safeguard clinical freedom and which built up its collective strength and identity within a dispersed professional group by perpetuating a myth that all GPs were equal. In fact, the developments were uneven, and during this time, the gap between the best and the worst GPs probably widened. The good GPs took advantage of the terms of the Charter, but those who did not choose to or who were denied opportunities to develop fell further and further behind. By the 1980s, there was an unacceptable degree of variation in general practice. This was not the diversity that is appropriate to small, community-based organizations responding to local needs. Instead, it was a lack of accountability and a failure of mechanisms to bring standards to the level of the best (Allsop, 1990).

The problems became most obvious in inner cities. In London in particular, the Acheson Report painted an unremittingly bleak picture of uncoordinated primary care services struggling to keep pace with demands (London Health Planning Consortium, 1981). One of the legacies of the report has been persistent pessimism about primary care in the capital, although measures were introduced that began to make the future look promising (Hughes and Gordon, 1992).

However, general practice development at the top end of the scale had also begun to falter. Even the good practices were pushing the Charter mechanisms to their limits. The cost–rent scheme, for example, was no longer a sufficient incentive to invest in premises when the price of property was rocketing. At this point, attention was deflected from the shortcomings of the system and turned instead to resisting the market-led reforms of the Thatcher administration.

General medical services are negotiated through a national contract with GPs; in 1990, this was revised (Department of Health, 1989a). The aim was to alter the clinical behaviour of GPs, introducing new clinics and targets. The contract created financial incentives for GPs to provide certain services, such as minor surgery and chronic disease management for asthma and diabetes, and encouraged increased participation in health promotion and prevention activities.

It proved to be very unpopular, and the long cycle of growing GP morale was shattered (Leese and Bosanquet, 1996).

Whatever its rights and wrongs, the contract was imposed on GPs and completely undermined their sense of being in control of progress. Progress was intertwined with their own personal aspirations in a way which was entirely understandable given the personal commitment many of them had made to putting general practice on the map. They saw themselves as moving from being champions of primary care to being servants of the new Family Health Services Authorities (FHSAs). They saw few additional rewards for good practice, but much additional bureaucracy.

Other commentators saw the rewards for preventive care in the new contract as progressive and supported the move towards some responsibility for the health of the whole practice population as well as for individual patients (Gillam et al, 1994). Deprivation payments were also seen as potentially beneficial, although, as they were not tied to performance, they created perverse incentives. However, there was a drastic downturn in GP morale. This had not been anticipated from what had been seen as a relatively limited reorganization of general medical service regulations. At a stroke, however, all the problems of general practice were laid at the door of the new contract (Leese and Bosanquet, 1996).

Fundholding was, and remains, the other major contentious issue within the profession, although the first waves of fundholding were largely built on *ad hoc* development by the entrepreneurial practitioners who had grasped the opportunities of the 1966 Charter. These are practices that are now able to operate as primary care organizations interacting with other organizations in the NHS. Fundholding has provided the opportunity for general practice as an organization, rather than GPs as individual professionals, to engage with the rest of the system (Plamping, 1995b).

GP fundholding was probably the most radical element of the 1990–91 NHS reforms. An internal market was created by encouraging hospitals to become self-governing provider Trusts, separated from district health authorities, and competing with each other for business. (Community Trusts, as discussed below, were not part of the initial thinking.) There were to be two kinds of purchaser: district health authorities and GP fundholders. Volunteer general practices were given funds to buy a range of hospital and community services for their patients. The BMA and most GPs were passionately against the scheme, but, despite early opposition, it has grown rapidly. By

1994, there were 1682 fundholding practices in England whose combined practice populations made up 36% of the population (in some places coverage being over 70%) (Coulter, 1995). Since then, even more interesting experiments in 'total fundholding' have been introduced, in which practices hold budgets for all their patients' health care needs, including accident and emergency, psychiatric in-patient and maternity care (National Health Service Executive, 1994; see also Chapter 2). These total fundholding schemes would appear to provide a much stronger incentive than does standard fundholding to provide primary care solutions to what are perceived as secondary care problems (Harrison and Choudhry, 1996). Fundholding as a method of allocating health services resources remains highly controversial:

> Its proponents claim that giving general practitioners control over budgets has resulted in improved efficiency, greater responsiveness to patients' needs and enhanced quality of care. Critics of the scheme argue that it leads to widening inequalities, fragmentation of services and deterioration in relationships with patients. (Coulter, 1995)

There are reports which show that fundholders believe they have achieved major benefits through the scheme, whilst similar claims are made by non-fundholding practices engaged in joint purchasing with local health authorities (Black et al, 1994; Glennerster et al, 1994).

The Conservative administration was confident of the success of fundholding (see National Health Service Executive, 1994). The Labour government favours locality commissioning, as highlighted in the 1997 White Paper (Secretary of State for Health, 1997). Either way, the focus for much of the 1990s has been on the role of GPs as purchasers of services and, thereby, the control mechanism for hospital referrals and costs. The role of GPs as providers of services has had rather less attention, although in a health service that aspires to become primary care led, the importance of general practice as the bedrock service provider can hardly be exaggerated. The policy emphasis is now moving in this direction with health authorities as commissioners of primary care services for local populations, something we return to later in this chapter and which is discussed in more detail in Chapter 2.

An historical perspective on community health services development

The community health services also moved a long way during the 1980s with the introduction of general management and their rescue from many years of neglect in the NHS policy world. Modern community health services are very diverse – some have grown out of hospital specialities, others are closely related to social care. The range of professional staff is wide, but nurses form the majority of the workforce. Modern nursing in the community comprises a vast range of skills and specialist as well as generalist knowledge, but the inherited traditions of community nursing go back a long way and help to explain the way in which the community health services have developed.

The roots of community nursing can be traced from the religious orders and charities of the Middle Ages, through the Poor Law committees with their parish nurses, to the reforming legislation of the late 19th and early 20th centuries. This established the basis for environmental health services between 1872 and 1875, registered midwives in 1902, founded a school health service in 1907 and a college of nursing in 1916, required home nursing for infectious disease in mothers and children in 1918, registered nurses in 1919 and reformed the professional body for home nurses into the Queen's Institute of District Nursing in 1925. When the Poor Law system ended in 1929, local authorities took over the responsibility for community nursing (Taylor, 1991).

The NHS Act in 1946 introduced a tripartite structure that preserved the separation of general practice, hospitals and community nursing and allied services. The most immediate changes came about in the hospital sector. Building on war-time emergency experience, private, charitable and local authority hospitals were brought together for the first time, to be managed under local and regional hospital committees. General practice was left to its own devices. Community health services were run by the local authorities. With notable exceptions, the medical officers of health of the local authorities did little to develop them (Beardshaw and Robinson, 1990). In the first major reorganization of the NHS in 1974, community services were removed from local authority control and combined with hospital services under new area health authorities, where they became the poor relations of the hospitals.

From the mid-1970s government policy began to give priority to developing the concept of 'community care'. Increasingly, emphasis was placed on the community health services but it was recognized that they suffered from lack of planning and were not organized to cope with the demands likely to be placed upon them. Within a few years, however, the community health services had begun to establish their own identity.

Patients First was the policy document that led to this and introduced ideas of consumerism and decentralization:

the closer decisions are taken to the local community and those who work directly with patients, the more likely it is that patients' needs will be their prime objective. ('Patients First' Consultation Paper, 1979)

The policy directive that followed suggested organizing community health services into discrete units of management, with the aim of giving them a single and authoritative voice. In the 1982 NHS reorganization, community units were created in most district health authorities (DHAs), followed by the creation of general management at district and then unit level. Many of these new general managers set about developing an explicit philosophy of community health service provision (Dalley, 1989).

On the nursing side, they were aided by two influential enquiries established in 1985 (Department of Health and Social Security, 1986; Welsh Office, 1988). Both documented the uneven development of community nursing, which in some places was quite clearly 'in a rut'. Both articulated a vision of neighbourhood nursing and primary care teams with skilled generalist nurses trained to assess local needs and provide individually tailored health care in or near people's homes. Changes began to be made at an unprecedented rate. With a responsibility to provide services to clearly defined populations, community services struggled to find ways of giving priority to disadvantaged groups such as homeless families, housebound elderly people and minority ethnic groups. Ambitious programmes of development were planned, and, with a growing sense of purpose, came higher visibility (Brown et al, 1988; Kalsi and Constantinides, 1989; Winn and Quick, 1990).

Policy-makers at regional and national level, however, were slow to improve their understanding of the contribution of community services to the health care system. At the point at which strategic decisions were being taken at the end of the 1980s, there was no clear idea of where the services were going or how they would relate to the other sectors. The policy document *Working for Patients* (Department of Health, 1989b) said a great deal about the directions that hospital and family practitioner services should take, but nothing about community health services. The NHS was to be reformed by making hospitals self-governing and GPs more competitive. In the field of community care – the 'other face' of the community health services – there was just as much uncertainty. The Griffiths report (Griffiths, 1988) recommended ways in which health and social services could work more effectively in practice to deliver government policy. However, the government's delay in responding to the report it had commissioned only added planning blight to confusion (Hughes, 1989).

In some perverse way, it seemed that just as the benefits of working for comprehensive community-based health care were becoming tangible, community units found themselves vulnerable to fragmentation and the fear that the most 'marketable' elements would have to link with hospitals or entrepreneurial general practices and the 'non-essential' services would be allowed to wither (Constantinides and Gordon, 1990; Haggard, 1990).

The Audit Commission reported and confirmed that, like general practice, community health services were unevenly developed across the country (Audit Commission, 1992). There was also another enquiry into nursing in the community (Roy, 1990). Following the 1990 NHS and Community Care Act, there was surprise and incomprehension within the Department of Health (DoH) when community units seized their opportunity and applied for Trust status in the 'first wave' procedures of the NHS reforms (Haggard, 1993). These procedures had been designed for hospitals, and 'in as much as there had been any thinking about the whole system it had been neatly parcelled up between general practice and hospitals' (Plamping, 1995c).

This over-simplified view has, however, been challenged. Some community Trusts are carving out a vigorous agenda for themselves (Bunce, 1993; Ellis, 1994). It is their capacity to deliver safe, high-quality care in or near people's homes that will determine much of the shift in services from hospital to community-based care, the so-called substitution agenda, in which not only the location of service, but also the type of professional delivering the service alters (Pedersen and Leese, 1997). However, the political climate at the end of the 1990s offers an uncertain environment in which there may be opportunities for innovation and market positioning but there are still 'many assumptions, prejudices, and vested interests blocking or imposing change' for community Trusts as providers of services (Office for Public Management, 1995). Trust mergers and new forms of primary care organization are on the cards. The boundary between health and social care continues to move. Community care reforms are the 'other' part of the 1990 NHS and Community Care Act, and securing integrated services to support vulnerable people in the community is an NHS priority. Joint commissioning initiatives between health and local authorities, for example, require greater co-ordination between home care and community nursing, and greater clarity about who does what in rehabilitation services (Poxton, 1996). The only certainty would seem to be that we can, over the next few years, expect many different models to emerge for the organization of community-based health services.

Pressures for change

The NHS is a complex, social institution, and, as such, we would expect it constantly to evolve and adapt. In recent years, powerful pressures for change have affected all industrialized nations who struggle with the problem of meeting health needs with finite resources (King's Fund Commission, 1992). These include the changing patterns of disease in industrialized nations, where chronic degenerative illnesses have become a major cause of ill-health and their management over time has become as important as the treatment of acute episodes. Life expectancy has risen, but with it has grown the tendency for longer periods of disabled living. Institutions are not geared to managing chronic illness, and health policy initiatives are turning instead towards emphasizing prevention and primary care.

Public attitudes are changing, as is our demography. We are living longer and producing fewer children. We are better informed and better educated than our grandparents, and we want to be more involved in the treatment choices made on our behalf. The choice of treatment is much greater than it was, and, for the most part, people want to be in hospital as little as possible.

Advances in technology mean that less invasive and more effective technical procedures reduce the length of time that patients need to stay in hospital, but may this may mean more time during which they need care at home. Many of the diagnostic, monitoring and treatment procedures that were previously only possible in hospital can now be carried out safely in people's homes.

Financial constraint, starting with the economic downturn of the mid-1970s, has led to a policy imperative of achieving control of public expenditure and getting value for money within the health sector.

In the UK, the Conservative government that came to power in 1979 promised a radical review of all aspects of the welfare state. The NHS was seen as inefficient, bureaucratic and resistant to change. The solution was to introduce working practices from the commercial world, in particular competition and consumerism. The NHS and Community Care Act 1990 introduced 'the reforms' at the core of which lay the purchaser/provider split, which brought market mechanisms to a publicly funded system. As highlighted earlier, health authorities, and some GPs, became purchasers of health services for their local populations. Hospitals and community units became provider Trusts, in competition for contracts. Some combined to offer both hospital and community services. Some GPs became fundholders, able to purchase hospital and community services on behalf of their patients. A complex annual process of negotiating contracts for services was put in place, and transaction costs rose.

In 1994, the NHSE introduced the rather ambiguous concept of a primary care-led NHS, discussed further in Chapter 2. GP fund-holding was seen as the principal mechanism behind the trend for more services to be provided in primary care settings. In 1996, health authorities and FHSAs were merged, and much of the hard-won experience of FHSA managers in developing primary care was lost.

The past decade has been a period of intense legislative activity, and the 1997 Primary Care Act looks set to influence primary care well into the next century. Implementation of this legislation will allow new kinds of primary care organization to emerge and could remove the GP monopoly on general medical services.

What next for primary care?

These latest reforms of the NHS are about the organization of primary care – who provides it, where it is provided, which professionals are involved and how they are trained. The reforms are about opening up the primary care 'market' to new providers. In their analysis of new arrangements, some of which will be piloted over the next few years, Coulter and Mays (1997) discuss the following:

- Health authorities could negotiate locally with general medical practices, and dental practices, for them to provide a range of specified services to meet the needs of local populations. These would be local whole-practice contracts rather than the national contract with individual practitioners as at present. Practices would employ other professionals, such as community nurses, therapists and specialists, on a sessional basis.
- Community Trusts and general practices might merge to form single, jointly managed organizations on contract to local health authorities.
- Health authorities might contract with a community Trust to provide all local primary care services. Trusts might employ salaried GPs and dentists, or sub-contract to selected practices.
- Acute Trusts might contract with a health authority to provide primary and secondary services, either the full range or selected services such as mental health.
- Consortiums of general practices in locality commissioning

groups or total fundholding groups could contract to provide the complete range of primary and secondary services.

In many ways, these proposals are a reflection of the numerous experimental models of primary care organization already being developed and tested around the country (Gordon and Hadley, 1996; Meads, 1996). Views are mixed about the likely impact of the legislation, some saying that it could lead to deregulation similar to that which hit the financial markets in 1986, others believing that it will bring minimal change because there is to be no compulsion and little incentive for professionals to form new organizations (Coulter and Mays, 1997)

Most commentators welcome these moves. They will allow a much wider choice in financing and contracting for general medical services. In the past, incentives have always been professionally targeted, for example GP fundholding or cost–rent schemes. In cities in particular, such national incentives have seldom worked as well as in other parts of the country, and improvements have not kept pace. The new arrangements make it possible for health authorities to contract with *the practice* (or other organization) *rather than the practitioner* and allow greater local flexibility to specify services that will meet local needs. This is surely a move in the right direction.

The commissioning of primary care services is a welcome shift in focus, but it is not at all clear that health authorities are in good shape to deliver. They are burdened with an annual contracting process and face increasing pressures to cut management costs. There is an important task in monitoring and regulating standards, but it is not yet clear how this will happen. Those health authority managers who currently work with general practice are mainly concerned with fundholding or commissioning groups purchasing other services. When health authorities merged with FHSAs in 1996, very few senior posts went to FHSA managers. One recent study shows that, of 87 health authority chief executives, only 7 have been FHSA general managers (Martin et al, 1997). What may have been lost is much of the experience of the enormously creative FHSA developments that went into general practices in recent years. General practices are highly varied, entrepreneurial, small-scale organizations that are not the same as hospitals or health authorities, and their scale matters if we want flexible, locally appropriate services. Yet the success of all the changes currently in the pipeline will depend to a greater or lesser extent on the willingness and consent of GPs at a time when the profession is questioning its role more than ever. Health authorities have a major task ahead, and although some are far advanced in their primary care strategies, others have a lot of catching up to do (Martin et al, 1997).

In general, patients are unlikely to notice much change, at least for the next few years. Most people will still go to their local surgery or health centre. They will still have the right to enrol with an NHS GP. The NHS will still be free at the point of delivery and will still be funded out of taxation. However, by the turn of the century, some people may have a greater choice of services: from a new primary care centre or a shopping centre or a hospital accident unit. They may have direct access to other health professionals, such as nurse practitioners or counsellors. They may have more access to specialist teams for asthma, for example, or mental health problems through so-called 'vertical integration' programmes. They may experience more co-ordination between health and social care, through 'primary managed care' programmes. Their experience of moving between home and hospital could improve through 'shared care' programmes. On the other hand, the risk is that services might become more impersonal and the one-to-one patient–doctor relationship weakened. For some, this relationship is a highly valued part of current primary care. For others, who may have had a different experience, the risk will be worth taking.

Conclusion

We may not be able to predict the impact of all the changes that have been put in motion, but we can identify some of the guiding principles for a commissioning strategy for primary care. These would allow us to ensure a greater consistency of standards while, at the same time, taking into account the distinctive qualities and the creativity and flexibility that are its strength. In summary, for the NHSE's key planning priority to succeed, primary care services should be:

- founded on the work of generalists, both doctors and nurses;
- supported by specialists;
- managed within a framework that ensures consistent quality;
- maintained at a scale appropriate to a personal care organization;
- able to manage chronic illness as an emergent condition rather than a series of events;
- able to combine person-centred care with population-based services.

References

Allsop J (1990) Changing Primary Care: The Role of Facilitators. London: King's Fund.

Audit Commission (1992) Homeward Bound: A New Course for Community Health. London: HMSO.

Balint M (1957) The Doctor, his Patient, and the Illness. London: Pitman Medical.

Beardshaw V, Robinson R (1990) New for Old? Prospects for Nursing in the 1990s. Research Report No. 8. London: King's Fund.

Black D, Birchall A D, Trimble I M G (1994) Non-fundholding in Nottingham: a vision of the future. British Medical Journal 309: 930–2.

Boufford J I (1994) Shifting the Balance from Acute to Community Health Care. London: King's Fund.

Brown P, Gordon P, Hughes J (1988) Changing School Health Services. London: King's Fund.

Bunce C (1993) Hospital at home is a feasible option. Fundholding 7: 14–16.

Constantinides P, Gordon P (1990) A model of service. Health Service Journal 100: 5222.

Coulter A (1995) General practice fundholding: time for a cool appraisal. British Journal of General Practice 45(392): 119–20.

Coulter A (1996) Why should health services be primary care led? Journal of Health Services Research Policy 1(2): 122.

Coulter A, Mays N (1997) Primary care: opportunities and threats. Deregulating primary care. British Medical Journal 314: 510–13.

Dalley G (1989) Community health services today. In Hughes J (Ed.) The Future of Community Health Services. London: King's Fund.

Department of Health (1989a) General Practice in the National Health Service. The 1990 Contract. London: HMSO.

Department of Health (1989b) Working for Patients. London: HMSO.

Department of Health and Social Security (1986) Neighbourhood Nursing: A Focus for Care. Chairman: Mrs Julia Cumberlege. London: HMSO.

Ellis N (1994) Community Health Services. Health News Briefing. London: Association of Community Health Councils of England and Wales.

Gillam S, McClenahan J, Plamping D, Harris J, Epstein C (1994) Community Oriented Primary Care. London: King's Fund.

Glennerster H, Matsaganis M, Owens P (1994) Implementing GP fundholding: wild card or winning hand? In Robinson R, Le Grand J (Eds) Evaluating the NHS Reforms. London: King's Fund.

Gordon P, Hadley J (Eds) (1996) Extending Primary Care – Polyclinics, Resource Centres, Hospitals at Home. Oxford: Radcliffe Medical Press.

Gordon P, Plamping D (1996) Primary health care - its characteristics and potential. In Gordon P, Plamping D (Eds) Extending Primary Care, Vol. 4. London: Radcliffe Medical Press/King's Fund.

Griffiths R (1988) Community Care: An Agenda for Action. London: HMSO

Haggard L (1990) A safety net for mending. Health Services Journal 100: 5223.

Haggard E (1993) Integrating primary and secondary care. In Cook H, Garside P (Eds) Managing NHS Trusts. Harlow: Longman.

Harrison S, Choudhry N (1996) General practice fundholding in the UK National Health Service: evidence to date. Journal of Public Health Policy 17(3): 331–46.

Heath I (1993) The future of general practice. In Lock S (Ed.) Eighty-five Not Out. London: King's Fund.

Hughes J (Ed.) (1989) The Future of Community Health Services. London: King's Fund.

Hughes J, Gordon P (1992) An Optimal Balance? Primary Health Care and Hospital Services in London. London Initiative Working Paper No. 8. London: King's Fund.

Kalsi N, Constantinides P (1989) Working towards Racial Equality in Health Care: The Haringey Experience. London: King's Fund.

King's Fund Commission (1992) London's Health Care in 2010. London: King's Fund.

Leese B, Bosanquet N (1996) Changes in general practice organisation: a survey of GPs' views on the 1990 contract and fundholding. British Journal of General Practice 46(403): 95–9.

London Health Planning Consortium (1981) Primary Health Care in Inner London. Report of a Studygroup. Chairman: E D Acheson. London: DHSS.

Martin D et al (1997) Who's sorry now? Health Service Journal (26 June): 28–30.

Meads G (1996) Future Options for General Practice. London: King's Fund/Radcliffe Medical Press.

Moore G T (1992) The disappearing generalist. Millbank Quarterly 70(2): 361–79.

National Health Service Executive (1994) Developing NHS Purchasing and General Practice Fundholding: Towards a Primary-care Led NHS. EL(94)79. London: NHSE.

National Health Service Executive (1995) Priorities and Planning Guidance for the NHS 1996/7. Leeds: NHSE.

Office for Public Management (1995) Beyond the Looking Glass: The Future for Community Trusts. London: Office for Public Management.

'Patients First' Consultation Paper (1979) Consultation Paper on the Structure and Management of the NHS in England and Wales. London: HMSO.

Pedersen L L, Leese B (1997) What will a primary care led NHS mean for GP workload? British Medical Journal 314: 1337–41.

Plamping D (1995a) Face-to-face with the next step: from general practice to primary care organisation. Primary Care Management 6(4): 3–8.

Plamping D (1995b) Putting Primary Care Centre Stage. NHS Handbook 10th Edn. Birmingham: NAHAT.

Plamping D (1995c) Solutions – but for which problems? In Anand P, McGuire P (Eds) Current Issues in the NHS: Implementing the Health Care Reforms. London: Stephen Rutt/Macmillan.

Poxton R (1996) Bridging the gap: joint commissioning of health and social care. In Harrison A (Ed.) Health Care UK 1995/6. London: King's Fund.

Pratt J (1995) Practitioners and Practices: A Conflict of Values? Oxford: Radcliffe Medical Press/King's Fund.

Roy S (1990) Nursing in the Community. London: NW Thames Regional Health Authority.

Royal College of General Practitioners (1972) The Future General Practitioner: Learning and Teaching. London: RCGP.

Secretary of State for Health (1997) The New NHS. London: HMSO.

Starfield B (1994) Is primary care essential? Lancet 344: 1129–33.

Starfield B (1995) Is strong primary care good for health outcomes? In Griffen J (Ed.) The Future of Primary Care. London: Office of Health Economics.

Taylor D (1991) Developing Primary Care. Opportunitites for the 1990s. Research Report No. 10. London: King's Fund.

Titmuss R M (1963) Essays on the Welfare State. London: Unwin University Books.

Welsh Office (1988) Nursing in the Community – a Team Approach for Wales. Chairman: Mrs Noreen Edwards. Cardiff: Welsh Office.

White K, Williams T F, Greenberg B G (1961) The ecology of medical care. New England Journal of Medicine 265: 885–92.

Winn K E, Quick A (1990) User Friendly Services. Guidelines for Managers of Community Health Services. London: King's Fund.

World Health Organisation (1978) Primary Health Care: Report of the International Conference on Primary Health Care, Alma-Ata, USSR 1978. Geneva: WHO.

Chapter 2
The organizational development of primary care

Geoff Meads

Context and purpose

As the previous chapter has illustrated, general medical practice has not only made a distinctive contribution to the NHS in the UK, but has also, in international terms, achieved a leading-edge status amongst alternative models of front-line primary health care services. Its unique combination of both high levels of professional training and competence, and public confidence – which do not always occur in a reciprocal relationship – together with the increasingly extended range of facilities sited in its surgeries and health centres, have served to consolidate its virtually unique position as gate-keeper to a country's entire health care system, both public and private. This position is historically derived from the basic philosophy of UK general practice: personal, comprehensive and continuous care. Over the past decade, the possible application of this holistic approach to issues of priority-setting has increasingly attracted attention. In particular, for those at national and local levels with both policy and operational responsibilities for NHS resource management, the pull has proved irresistible. Given a more flexible organizational framework that releases UK primary care from its reliance on uni-professional monopolies, the prize at stake has quite simply been the control and maintenance of a viable health care system.

The outcome has been primary care-led purchasing, the umbrella term afforded to the recent local arrangements, mostly within individual practices or clusters of practices, that have arisen as a result of the deliberate convergence of NHS clinical referral powers, service development responsibilities and financial controls throughout the local settings of primary care. In 1998, it is no longer enough for a GP to be simply a demand-led service provider for individuals and fami-

21

lies, however capable, respected or indeed rooted he, or increasingly she, may be in this role. Planning and contracting responsibilities now come with the job. In the language of the post-1997 new Labour administration, 'Primary Care Commissioning' is a universal given factor.

This broadening of the relationship between general practice and its external environment has significant implications for the wider organizational development of primary care in the UK. In particular, the concept of partnership and its expression is being redefined. The overall trend is away from organizational structures and processes based on control by a uni-disciplinary monopoly, that is, GPs, to more participative forms of leadership in team- or network-based enterprises that demonstrate increasing levels of cross-sector collaboration and interprofessional involvement, which will be discussed further in the following chapters. General practice has found itself, within a relatively short period, with a much larger number of interested parties and genuine stakeholders.

The increasing visibility of general practice has brought a growing awareness of the anachronism that is the legal partnership as the exclusive form of organizational status for medical practice in primary care. Moreover, as alternative types of primary care organization begin to emerge, the traditional assumptions about the efficacy of that practice itself are increasingly being questioned. In global terms, the British GP may have been seen as something special, but by international standards, the shortfalls are also all too evident. Figure 2.1 sets out a summary of the WHO's policy criteria for primary care, and it is readily apparent that in three out of the eight specified components at least, UK general practice has been fundamentally deficient. Figure 2.2 builds on the work of Professor Patrick Pietroni at the Marylebone

1.	Health education*
2.	Proper nutrition*
3.	Basic sanitation including safe water*
4.	Maternal and child health care
5.	Comprehensive immunization
6.	Prevention and control of endemic disease
7.	Treatment of basic health condition
8.	Satisfactory supply of drugs

*Indicates those areas traditionally outside the direct remit of UK general practice.

Figure 2.1: Primary health care: the core components
Source: World Health Organisation (1978).

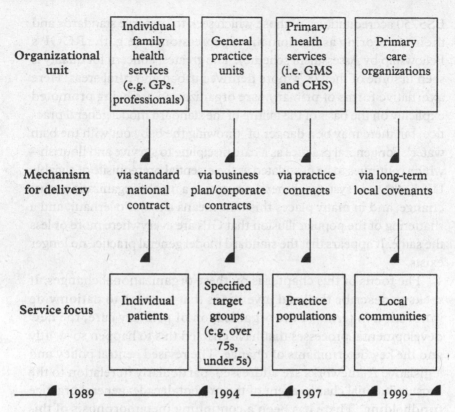

Organizational unit	Individual family health services (e.g. GPs. professionals)	General practice units	Primary health services (i.e. GMS and CHS)	Primary care organizations
Mechanism for delivery	via standard national contract	via business plan/corporate contracts	via practice contracts	via long-term local covenants
Service focus	Individual patients	Specified target groups (e.g. over 75s, under 5s)	Practice populations	Local communities
	1989	1994	1997	1999

Figure 2.2: UK policy for primary care 1989–99
Source: Adapted from Pietroni and Pietroni (1996).
GMS = General Medical Services; CHS = Community Health Services.

Centre (Pietroni and Pietroni, 1996) and distills the direction of travel in terms of UK policy in the 1990s. The increasing alignment with the WHO's framework is evident. Until now, since the inception of the NHS, general practice has been almost unquestioningly accepted in the UK as being synonymous with primary care, and top-quality primary care at that. For growing numbers of observers and patients, such assertions are beginning to sound hollow.

The theme of the President of the General Medical Council, Sir Donald Irvine, that general practice will continue to be the bedrock of the NHS but only if it addresses the increasingly visible local and nationwide variations in its quality (Irvine and Irvine, 1996), has led rapidly to at least six major practice accreditation programmes becoming available across the UK (Holden and Spooner, 1997). These programmes range from those which focus on the practice as an organization newly accessible to external review (e.g. the King's Fund Organisational Audit programme or British Standards Institution

BS5750 accreditation), to those which seek to preserve standards and
their monitoring as the domain of professionals (e.g. the RCGP's
Fellowship by Assessment scheme). The greatest concern for quality is
seen in some of the UK's more deprived urban and rural areas. Here
alternative forms of primary care organization are being promoted
explicitly on the basis of the failure of the standard model general practice, but there may be a danger of 'throwing the baby out with the bath
water'. For general practice as a care discipline to survive and flourish –
which continues to be postulated as the essential prerequisite of a viable
UK health care system – general practice as a unit of organization must
change, and in many places this now means a major overhaul, and a
shattering of the popular illusion that GPs are everywhere more or less
the same. It appears that the standard model general practice no longer
exists.

The focus of this chapter is on these organizational changes. It
seeks to describe the local inventions that have led to nationwide
innovation in terms of the organization of primary care, the new
developmental processes that have enabled this to happen so swiftly
and the key determinants of change. The revised central policy and
legislative frameworks are addressed, particularly in relation to the
most influential change agent of the present decade: general practice
fundholding. There has been a continuing metamorphosis of this
scheme as its remit has extended from being perceived as an end in
itself to becoming the means of something quite different: the local
ownership of a reconstituted and regenerated NHS. Curiously, within the contemporary version of the localized NHS, provider deregulation in primary care is now considered to be as important for
bonding purposes, as the single, uniform national contract for GPs
was to the pre-1990s NHS. Local diversity and devolution have
become new relational trademarks around which the tensions
between competition and collaboration will have to be resolved.
Primary care and its new organizations are the vehicle through which
the bureaucratic institution of the old NHS is not only translating
itself into the wider UK health care system, but also ensuring that the
public–private alliances, coalitions and the inter-relationships that
characterize the latter identify themselves within the contemporary
meaning of the NHS. The challenge, of course, is that they do so as
real stakeholders, with a full commitment and sense of belonging.
This is what Etzioni has described as the modern 'Spirit of
Community', embracing all sectors and characterized by the 'norma-
tive integration' that he was once only able to attribute empirically to
public service organizations (Etzioni, 1961, 1995).

Primary care-led purchasing

This term originated in the Wessex NHS Region in 1992/93. As Figure 2.3 illustrates, it was one of five strategic themes presented by the then Wessex Regional Health Authority, designed to take forward its overall objective of making 'primary care the principal focus of responsibility for health and health care'. However, it was not the first theme, nor was it another term for general practice fundholding. Indeed, it was originally applied at least as much to individual DHAs and the integrated DHAs/FHSAs 'health commissions' serving as the combined management agencies in 1992/93. Primary care-led purchasing, in the Wessex stratagey, was the stage a practice reached when it had developed consciously into a provider, that is, where the services supplied were demonstrably cost- and clinically effective, and inter-professionally resourced and supported, with the clear prospect of being able actively to engage individually and collectively with local people in the determination of present and future priorities (see Aim 4 in Figure 2.3). It predicated a maturity in the participating general practices that was not a prerequisite nationally. This motivation was not bought cheaply. Local DHAs such as Dorset transferred annual revenue sums of between £10 million and £20 million to ensure that practices had viable mid-term health targets and organizational development plans. They thereby paved the way for primary care to enter the

---

Strategic Objective:
To develop Primary Care as the Principal Focus of Responsibility for Health and Health Care.

Specific Aims:
1. To promote service investment in primary care wherever both clinically and cost effective
2. To extend the Primary Care Team as the basic service unit in the community
3. To encourage inter-professional partnerships, particularly in education and training
4. To move towards comprehensive Primary Care-led Purchasing through appropriate local organisational models
5. To ensure patients participate fully throughout the planning, provision and review stages of services and their treatment

---

Figure 2.3: Wessex Regional Health Authority: strategic themes
Source: Wessex Regional Health Authority (September 1993).

commissioning arena, addressing health purchasing as well as health care needs, both long and short term, across care sectors with responsibility for local populations rather than just individual patients. Wessex was the first part of the country to move beyond simply contracting for improved control or purchasing for greater efficiency of secondary care.

In contrast with this regional perspective, general practice fund-holding nationally during the first half of the 1990s rapidly became a first-order initiative in terms of central policy. Its accelerated implementation was an absolute political imperative, circumventing the preconditions of primary care development set out in the Wessex model. Introduced in 1990/91 by the then Secretary of State, Kenneth Clarke, with the expressed aim of reaching a final population coverage of around 6%, by 1997/98 the actual figure for fund-holding had risen to over 60%, with such districts as Wakefield and the Isle of Wight being almost completely fundholder covered. This dramatic shift in the role of fundholding from the 'gingering-up', through a degree of local competition, of the purchasing function of DHAs, to becoming the preferred vehicle for putting the emerging concept of commissioning into practice was most apparent in central NHS policy communications such as EL(94)79 (National Health Service Executive, 1994).

In 1993, the then Minister for Health, Brian Mawhinney, forcefully set out the government's commitment to the purchasing function. His 'Six Steps' were targeted overwhelmingly at health authorities, whose members were then briefed on the relevant central directives around the country. By October 1994, the impetus of fundholding was such that the policy direction was already fundamentally changing. It would become the health authorities' role to advise and support GPs in their purchasing responsibilities, and not vice versa as had hitherto been the case (National Health Service Executive, 1994).

In short, the UK was moving 'Towards a Primary Care-Led NHS', and this heading was immediately adopted into successive statements of NHS *Medium Term Planning Priorities and Annual Objectives*. Figure 2.4 displays the relevant extract from the 1996/97 version. A primary care-led NHS had quickly become the first of just six national priorities, and fundholding expansion was the chief objective. It was a remarkable move, which, not surprisingly, attracted considerable interest abroad and controversy at home. In terms of the organizational development of primary care, it meant that the UK remained very much the front-runner. For the NHS

Priority A. Work towards the development of a primary care-led NHS, in which decisions about the purchasing and provision of health care are taken as close to patients as possible.

Milestones

A1. There should be demonstrable progress in developing partnerships between health authorities and GPs, particularly through implementation of the national framework for GP fundholder accountability and development programmes for primary health care teams and health authority staff.

A2. Each Health Authority should have secured agreement to a local strategy for health and service improvement reflecting the objectives of 'The Health of the Nation', developed in partnership with GPs locally, other agencies and through consultation with local people.

A3. There should be measurable progress in reshaping traditional patterns of service to achieve an appropriate balance, between hospital and community provision, reflecting both patients' preferences to be treated at home or in their own community, and the need for certain services to be concentrated to secure effective clinical outcomes.

A4. Each Health Authority should have demonstrated a significant increase in the numbers of GPs directly involved in purchasing, particularly through the expanded fundholding options.

Figure 2.4: 1996/97 NHS medium-term priorities
Source: National Health Service Executive (1995).

itself, the impact upon the *status quo* was such that its million employees often seemed like ambassadors for uncertainty as they struggled to come to terms with what the changes could mean for their own roles and responsibilities (Fritchie, personal communication, 1997).

The label of a 'primary care-led NHS' clearly had its origins in the term coined in the Wessex region of 'primary care-led purchasing'. The respective impacts of these terms were, however, fundamentally different. Whereas the group of leading professional practitioner representatives, local health authority Directors of Primary Care and regional health authority (RHA) members that met in Winchester were concerned to find a phrase that bridged the gap between fundholders and non-fundholding GPs, and to create a common cause with the newly created health commissions, their counterparts in Leeds and London were geographically closer to central government departments, with the result that the words 'Towards a Primary Care-Led NHS' very quickly assumed political connotations. The NHS was seen as being defined in relation to the power of one of its constituents (over the rest). For those who were direct employees of the NHS, the effect in many places, particularly those where the quality of general practice was inadequate, was to engender downright alienation and hostility. That GPs with their independent contractor status could be legitimately regarded as partially detached from the NHS or, even worse, as the vanguard of the independent sector paving the way for ultimate privatization clearly for many spelt disaster. Privatization, hugely ill defined in its meaning, became by the mid-1990s the bogeyman for the organizational development of the whole NHS.

The cohesion and coherence that lay behind the concept of primary care-led purchasing was, as a consequence, manifestly in danger of being lost. At its inception, the term was deliberately not associated solely with GPs. It was, however, explicitly associated with a strengthening of public health, through the incorporation of data from local primary care settings into needs assessment and commissioning priorities. This meant placing issues of, for example, back pain, stress, chronic disease, handicap and patient transport alongside such Health of the Nation targets as cancer, stroke and coronary heart disease reduction. Individual patient and general population dimensions were thus entwined. Fortunately, the phrase not only became popular in Wessex – being recognized by over 70% of staff in internally commissioned staff feedback surveys at the time – but also led to tangible products in terms of both services and structures. Alternative primary care organizations began incrementally but steadily not only to develop, but also, through their entrepreneurial leadership, to lobby for fundamental changes in national policy and regulations to remove the plethora of centrally determined contractual restraints on their freedom and growth. Primary managed care was conceived.

New primary care organizations

Primary managed care was a concept introduced into the NHS lexicon by perhaps the UK's most influential local GP in the early 1990s, Dr Barry Robinson, from Lyme Regis. Here, on the borders of Dorset and Devon, in geographical terms virtually cut off by the Purbeck Hills from the mainland and with a largely retired, elderly practice population, Dr Robinson, with the support then of local GPs, other professionals and, crucially, the local people themselves, created the Lyme Regis Community Care Company in 1992/93. Although not a fundholding operation, it encapsulated the essential philosophy of primary care-led purchasing, functioning as if in the local ownership of the practice population, which, because of the geographical location of Lyme Regis, is virtually conterminous with the boundaries of the local community. Geographical and relational boundaries are in an unusual alignment. Well documented elswhere (Robinson, 1993, 1994), the company rapidly gained the confidence of both the local Dorset Health Authority and an initially hesitant Dorset County Council Social Services Department, to such an extent that, by 1995/96, it was directly managing virtually the whole of their combined resource allocation for the local population. The result was a substantial decline in institutional referrals and ten new provider contracts for such services as hospital-at-home, community nursing and physiotherapy lodged with the Community Care Company.

This venture represented not simply a triumph of individual local intervention in the context of a sympathetic national policy context. Intellectually, managed care as a theoretical construct was also increasingly taking root, translating itself from its US health maintenance organization origins into the evidence-based medicine movement of the UK, which is now, as Muir Gray has recently illustrated, crucially dependent upon primary care endorsement for its effective impact. Muir Gray recognizes the challenge that this involves in moving from patient- to disease-based management systems, subject to standard guidelines with set incentives and sources of provision (Muir Gray, 1997). For this to become primary managed care in the UK context today, of course, general practice still has to have direct control of both significant providing and purchasing functions.

Lyme Regis and its growing number of counterparts in the mid-1990s signified a fundamental shift from condition-specific clinical disciplines to the overall needs of individuals as the service focus in primary care, with the associated new responsibility for managing on behalf of the NHS the albeit limited resources available through the settings of modern general practice. This was an historic development, with important implications not least for role differentiation between and within professional groups. Primary managed care can be seen to have led, on the one hand, to the advent of nurse practitioners (see Chapter 3) and what some observers identify as a long-term trend to more generic community nursing (Bagnall and Gardner, 1997). In addition, it influenced a decline in that persisting NHS belief – the existence of nationwide equivalence in the standard of GP services. The King's Fund Development Centre team has led the way in distinguishing between the different family physicians, health care shapers and commissioning chief executives who now

populate the UK primary care scene (Plamping, 1995), for whom
the common denominator is increasingly being reduced to the length
and structure of their GP training. Figure 2.5 outlines the different
GP roles that can be identified in the second half of the 1990s, with
the parallel role developments for health authorities, which are facing
similar pressures to rationalize and refine their functions as a result of
the primary care-led NHS.

As Figure 2.5 illustrates, this new range of roles had developed in
tandem with the new diversity of primary care organizations. The
effective implementation of primary managed care had depended
upon the successful devolution of responsibilities previously retained
at intermediate or even central levels in the NHS: clinical effectiveness protocols, differential funding allocations, priority-setting and
joint service-planning. This devolution has permitted the emergence
of the organizational variants that are summarized in Table 2.1. Each
fits its local circumstances. Finding a label is the last task. The purpose and the population characteristics are paramount in deciding
management arrangements and then, finally, the title of the new primary care organizations. The East Southampton Community
Development Agency began, for example, with a deep concern for
urban decline and its consequences, and a need to counter the
resource-consuming tendencies of a local major teaching hospital.
Elsewhere, the Isle of Wight consortium model, designed by Dr Hugh
Maclean, was the more appropriate organizational development. A
single collective strength was essential if the county council was to be
persuaded of the case for conterminosity with the front-line NHS in
the joint provision of a range of community services. In Stroud, the
heady mixture of complementary therapies, New Age activists and
old-style Conservatism meant that pastoral care was the theme. To
date, each primary care organization has been a local creature and a
local creation.

Individually, several of these new models seem likely to survive
and succeed; some will probably not. Small individual total fundholding practices, for example, could well become defunct under the
present Labour government, which prefers primary or locality commissioning approaches, where from their perspective organizational
units have sufficient critical mass to merit the alignment of an NHS
planning and providing responsibilities in primary care. At the time
of writing, the jury remains out as to whether or not UK general practice collectively can respond to the changes in the political environment with sufficient rigour and flexibility to retain at least a large part
of its previous monopoly position. The individual entrepreneurial

GP type	HA type	Service focus	Typical location	Primary care organization type
A. Patient advocate/ activist	Development agency	Under performance	Deprived inner city	Primary care NHS Trust/GP advisory forums
B. Individual family/ physician	Contracts monitor	Medical treatment	Suburbs	Extended general practices/primary health care teams
C. Care co-ordinator/ manager	Co-purchaser	Seamless care	Market town	Community or pastoral care centres
D. Health care shaper/ commissioning executive	Regulator	Health/health care programmes	Random	Consortia/locality commissioning groups

Figure 2.5: An NHS focused on primary care: emerging roles, 1995–2000

Table 2.1: Primary care organizational developments

Role Type (source)	Purpose	Management	Population
1. The managed practice (e.g. Portsmouth)	Provider of standard Family and Community Health Services	Senior practitioner-led GP partnership operating to locally negotiated contract with HA for national 'core' services; employer of community nurses	2000 × 5 plus; universal, based on current distribution of GPs
2. The total fundholder (e.g. Runcorn)	Comprehensive commissioning of health care for individual practice population	GP partnership including managing partner with full activity based and benchmark budget	10,000–60,000; universal, some rationalization of service outlets
3. The preferred provider (e.g. Winchester)	Transfer of secondary care to community settings under GP control	Locality GP group through which one HA accredited practice purchases on behalf of neighbouring practices and employs or contracts for range of clinicians and CHS	40,000–80,000; large towns without full DGHs and range of premises available
4. The consortium (e.g. Isle of Wight)	Effective joint planning and provision of services with health and local authorities	Steering group of individual general practice representatives, with finance and development support staff and range of GPFH/GMS allocations at individual practice levels	50,000–100,000; local community with clear boundaries
5. The primary care agency (e.g. Andover)	Pooling of local purchaser and provider allocations to integrate and extend primary care	Executive agency under contract to local community trust and GPFHs with overall budgetary and service co-ordination responsibilities	50,000–100,000; overspill urban areas

(contd)

Table 2.1: (contd)

Role Type (source)	Purpose	Management	Population
6. The community development agency (e.g. East Southampton)	Maximize and protect primary health care services contribution in local areas with significant social and economic needs	GP co-operative with multi-fund arrangements and shared out-of-hours rotas and information network	50,000–100,000; inner city areas, counterpart to large DGH
7. The pastoral care centre (e.g. Stroud)	Promotion of individual citizen's and community health through combined medical and spiritual focus	Charitable status with user forums supporting range of complementary therapies	Under 10,000; universal but not discrete to localities
8. The community care centre (e.g. Yaxley)	Provide a major unified resource for information, support and advice to exploit local potential for community self-help	Centre management group includes user representatives with strong Patients Association; integrated GPFH and SSD care management budgets, and proprietary links to local residential and day care units	10,000–25,000; small towns, suburbs with single large established general practices
9. The primary care Trust (e.g. Peterborough)	Community-based provider control of local NHS resources and strategy augmented by private finance	Merged general practices and community trust as independent organization along 'golf club' lines with range of membership options and board of stakeholder representatives	100,000 plus; urban areas where GMS under-developed and limited premises available

(contd)

Table 2.1: (contd)

Role Type (source)	Purpose	Management	Population
10. The joint venture (e.g. Minehead)	Successful business development of general practices and private enterprises in the public interest	Extended partnerships, with commercial associates and alliances including retail pharmacies	10,000 plus; universal, but in areas where non-NHS services by patient payment viable
11. The primary managed care organization (e.g. Lyme Regis)	Transfer of health and health care responsibilities to the individual	Not for profit limited company, with patients as subscribers, comprehensive local financial allocation and contracting responsibilities delegated from HA, and local consultation on service priorities	10,000 plus; established local communities with strong general practice affiliations

CHS = community health services; DGH = district general hospital; HA = health authority; GMS = general medical services; GPFH = general practice fundholding; SSD = social services department.
Source: Meads (1996).

leadership of GPs that is represented by Table 2.1 is by no means universal. General practice is not everywhere the master of its own destiny, particularly not in the country's more deprived urban areas. Systematic evaluation, principally through action research, is clearly an essential requirement for the new organizational developments in primary care, and, under Professor David Wilkins' leadership, this approach already figures prominently in the agenda and output of the recently established National Primary Care Research and Development Centre in Manchester (NPCRDC; National Primary Care Research and Development Centre, 1997).

The NPCRDC expects to offer an important focus for understanding the future practice and policy implications of the 1997 Primary Care Act, which has effectively legitimized, through central statute, the translation of the separate professional family health services into the interdisciplinary primary care organizations of the future. Initiated by the previous Conservative government during Stephen Dorrell's tenure as Secretary of State, the Act was inherited by the new Minister for Health with responsibility for Primary Care, Alan Milburn, in May 1997. Although the new government quickly set about dismantling many aspects of the previous government's NHS internal market (National Health Service Executive, 1997), this legislation remained virtually untouched. Around 600 applications to be local pilot sites for alternative organizational status were, accordingly, still encouraged. The originating Bill passed through its parliamentary committee stages at a remarkable rate during the hectic, pre-general election months of early 1997. It garnered all-party support with singular ease. The dividends of new organizational developments in primary care attracted a tacit political consensus amongst those exercising the overall collective responsibility for health care in the UK. This support mirrored that gained by the pre-legislation year-long 'listening exercise' undertaken nationwide in 1995/96 right across the NHS by Stephen Dorrell himself, and his then Minister of Health, Gerald Malone, which led to the consultative document on the future of primary care (Secretary of State for Health, 1996a), in which local flexibility and alternative organizational developments were first officially flagged up for central government action.

The value-for-money potential of larger and fewer front-line services, increasingly set up as joint ventures in terms of their income and investment streams, with patients themselves helping to determine less expensive and professionally defensive skills mixes, is simply a prospect too good to miss. Also, these dividends are not so much a future bonus as an imminent necessity: extended primary health services must take on an altogether more prominent role in a contemporary NHS that has effectively capped its institutional capacity through the combination of long-stay hospital replacement programmes, the reprofiling of many acute elective admissions into day care procedures and the withdrawal (post-1993) from direct nursing home provision.

The 1997 Primary Care Act offered, via national pilot site status, four routes to organizational diversity in primary care (Secretary of State for Health, 1996b). In summary these are:

1. A supplementary contract to augment at practice level the national general medical services contract for individual general medical practitioners, to supply additional services funded through a health authority's hospital and community health services financial allocations.

2. A combined general medical services and community health services agreement enabling the practice to become a primary care organization directly responsible for integrated community services (e.g. nursing and paramedical support).
3. A fully funded practice population-based contract with virtually the total NHS allocation attached, levied in accordance with general medical services and hospital and community health services weighted capitation criteria.
4. Access to NHS contracts for all family health services contractors, including in particular general dental practitioners and community pharmacists, regardless of geographical boundaries, for services not currently covered by NHS statutory regulations.

Each of the above has proved attractive, and although the independent sector has been explicitly excluded from a direct role in actual service provision, at least at the early stage of development, which coincides with the publication of this book, other forms of stakeholding (e.g. capital investment, facilities and management) have been encouraged; health parks (e.g. Bristol and Gloucester) and resource centres (e.g. Wakefield, Enfield and Haringey) being the most visible expressions of these emerging joint ventures.

New primary care organizations and the mixed economy of community care and its funding are self-evidently synonymous. If primary care cannot pay effectively for secondary care, who pays for primary care and its development? This seems likely to be an increasingly demanding question for those with policy responsibilities at both local and national levels in the not-so-distant future.

Contemporary NHS development

The changing organizations of primary care have been the vehicle through which, during the 1990s, the institution of the NHS has translated itself into the wider UK health care environment. Their emergence, and the ways in which they have emerged, have helped to determine a fundamental set of changes in the way in which the NHS itself develops. The result is that the NHS itself, as it approaches the millennium, is a very different type of organization from that of a decade ago. While politicians of all parties decry its excessive bureaucracy – by which they usually mean its administrative overhead – the NHS has, in theoretical terms, actually shed many of the characteristics of a classic bureaucratic organization (Meads, 1997).

As Professor Ham's diagram (Figure 2.6) illustrates, even as late as 1992 it was tenable to depict the NHS as a conventional command-and-control hierarchy. The primary care-led NHS ended all of that, with over 400 statutory NHS organizations being terminated in the first half of the present decade. The new Labour government soon discovered that the challenge that it inherited of re-integrating the NHS required an essentially process-oriented relational response, given that standard structural solutions of organizational re-engineering were no longer to hand. The membership of the NHS has changed. It now belongs to stakeholders rather than just employees, to sub-contractors as well as professionals, and, perhaps in the future, to individual patients as well as the body politic. The theoretical constructs that now apply are those of organizational psychologists and sociologists drawn from the world of US corporations or international conglomerates, where, over the past 30 years, the organization has been defined as a coalition of groups and sub-groups, in which

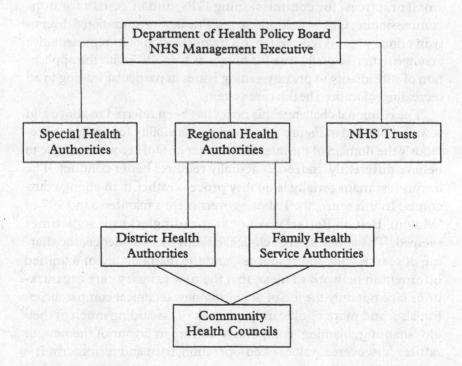

Figure 2.6: The structure of the NHS after 1990
Source: Ham (1992).

'organic adaptive' survival is defined as success, and where central leadership is signified by strategic concepts steering overall performance calculated merely as the sum of the separate parts (Cyert and March, 1963; Argyris, 1964; Bennis, 1966).

It is primary care organizational development that, above all, has paved the way for this transformation. GPs remain independent contractors – private sector businessmen. They own their partnerships. They operate to their own annual business plans, rendering redundant, as primary care-led purchasers, the detailed 5- and 10-year individual service plans so characteristic of RHAs and DHAs prior to 1990. They exercise power chiefly through the informal organization of the NHS and are themselves most significantly influenced by peer pressures. Difference is legitimate, and the traditional NHS value of equality has become first equity and then equivalence. The need to justify this variety and yet still suggest the respectability of self-regulating quality has been paramount, hence the plethora of primary care associations in the 1990s. These are no longer just the umbrella national organizations of the General Medical Services Committee and RCGP but a whole range of associations: for fundholding GPs, for multi-funds, for small practices, for commissioning GPs, and of course for non-commissioning GPs as well, and so on. The new organizational diversity in primary care is reflected in this fragmentation of its representative arrangements – equally true for nurses as for GPs – with the application of subsidiarity to priority-setting issues in particular leading to an increasingly localized health care system.

The relational challenge this poses has been referred to above and is well illustrated in Figure 2.7. Local responsibility for decisions previously the domain of the intermediate tier or DoH requires people to behave differently. Indeed, it actually requires better conduct. The litmus test managerially is quality process rather than change outcomes. In this sense, the Labour government's manifesto in 1997 of 'Making Britain Better' was not as meaningless as it sometimes seemed. The application of clinical effectiveness evidence, the sharing of scarce skills and resources, and the membership of a unified information network all mean that the new primary care organizations face not only the job of acquiring new technical competencies, but also, and more significantly, the task of discarding much of their old 'shaming, blaming' competitive culture in favour of the new, or rather rediscovered, values of co-operation, trust and reciprocity. It is a formidable challenge and represented for some professionals in UK primary care a complete change of direction. For the majority, however, it is, at the time of writing, a reassurance and a relief.

A. Pre-1990s: Familial
    Parent ——▶ Child   e.g. Consultants to patients, DHA to CHC
    Child ——▶ Parent   e.g. NHS to Department of Health, FHS
                            Contractors to FHSA/FPC (pre-1990
                            family practitioner committee)

B. 1990–96: Immature/transitional
    Child ——▶ Adult   e.g. HAs in deficit with NHSE regional
                            offices, new PCTs with HAs
    Adult ——▶ Parent   e.g. NHS Trusts with HAs, NHSE with DoH

C. Post-1997 (?): Mature prospective
    Adult ——▶ Adult   e.g. HA/GPFH strategic alliances, preferred
                            provider long-term service agreements, RO
                            market regulation, GP–patient priority-setting

Figure 2.7: The NHS relationships set. DHA = district health authority; CHC = community health council; FHSA = family health services authority; FPC = family practitioner committee; HA = health authority; NHSE = National Health Service Executive; PCT = primary care team; DoH = Department of Health; CPFH = GP fundholding; RO = Regional Office of the National Health Service Executive.
Reproduced by kind permission of Radcliffe Medical Press.
Source: Meads (1997).

Conclusion

The structures of primary care in the UK, and with them the relationships between front-line professionals in the community, have been transformed by the policy initiatives of the early and mid-1990s, and transformed irrevocably. A 'primary care-led NHS', by whatever name it may acquire in the future, is here to stay. The sustenance and survival of the NHS, within the framework of a society in which democracy increasingly demands a combination of elected, appointed and, above all, individual consumerist sources of legitimacy for public service decision-making – and at ever more localized levels – requires significant participation and effectively managed implementation if processes founded upon the principle of subsidiarity are to endure. Emerging primary care organizations are an expression of these trends. Primary care-led purchasing, at its very different stages of local development according to the differing local conditions, as Figure 2.8 indicates, is now a core responsibility of these organizations. The selective private sector US health maintenance organization has traditionally been an anathema to the UK GP seeing himself propping up a general taxation-funded, free-for-all, universal NHS.

Steps
1 Input from individual practices to commissioning priorities.
2 Input from groups of general practices representative of a district to
   its purchasing decisions.
3 Combinations of local primary health care teams (PHCTs) coming
   together to influence health authority decisions.
4 Local PHCTs compiling individual health plans for submission to
   the health authority to influence purchasing decisions.
5 Combinations of local PHCTs compiling one unified health plan to
   influence purchasing decisions.
6 Individual PHCTs compiling a health plan and being allocated
   indicative budgets by the health authority, but with purchasing still
   undertaken by the latter.
7 Combinations of local PHCTs compiling a health plan to influence
   purchasing decisions and bidding for contracts for shared services.
8 Individual PHCTs or groups of PHCTs compiling a local health plan
   and receiving allocations for the purchase and provision of agreed
   services.
9 Combinations of local PHCTs compiling a local health plan and
   social care plan and receiving allocations from the health authority
   for the purchase and provision of agreed services. Staff may be
   employed within the PHCTs as care managers with a limited budget
   for social care.
10 Combinations of local PHCTs compiling a local health plan and
   social care plan and being commissioned by the health authority and
   social services department for the purchase and provision of agreed
   health and social care programmes.

Figure 2.8: Levels of primary care-led purchasing: climbing the ladder
Source: Adapted from Meads (1996).

They now increasingly have much in common, and tomorrow's GP
may well see his support role to the wider health care system being
dependent on the size and security of the salary that his primary
managed care enterprise or company can offer.

Strategic developments in the contemporary NHS are essentially
emergent and processual. They require retrospective understanding
rather than rational explanation. The diffuse nature of UK general
practice, allied to its new powers of resource utilization, reinforce this
perspective and will continue to do so. The key policy questions for
the future organizational development of primary care are not difficult to deduce. How will patients themselves legitimize the new primary care organizations? What will be the frameworks for more
efficient combinations of health and social services in primary care?
How will their effectiveness be assessed? What forms will accreditation and regulation assume?

Those who have crafted the policies that have shaped the organizational developments in primary care have, in effect, worked to a 70% success rule. They have recognized that they are operating in a health care environment in which there is a new direct relationship between the DoH and its primary care units (McKeon, 1996). The traditional intervening levels (e.g. RHAs and Family Practitioner Committees) are no longer there. The direct central/local dynamic is powerful, productive but often unpredictable. It has led, for example, to the advent of 24-hour, out-of-hours co-operatives seemingly almost overnight across the country. On the other hand, emergency referral rate increases continue unabated and seemingly unconstrained by the GPs' influence over their patients. For policy-makers, today's NHS is virgin territory. There are no maps to follow and few reference points: in terms of designing and developing health care systems, nobody has been there before.

In such circumstances, policy deliberately leaves 30% of the agenda for another time, for local solutions to start to emerge. Also, 20% of the 70% can be expected to turn out not quite as expected. So it is for future organizational developments in primary care. The story, it seems, started by the GP entrepreneurs whose new ventures and writings (Meads, 1995) broke the mould of partnership in 1995, has still only just begun.

References

Argyris C (1964) Integrating the Individual and the Organisation. New York: John Wiley & Sons.

Bagnall P, Gardner L (1997) Primary Care Nursing: Managing the Journey Ahead. London: Queen's Nursing Institute.

Bennis W G (1966) Organisational developments and the fate of bureaucracy. Industrial Management Review 7: 41–55.

Cyert R, March J (1963) A Behavioural Theory of the Firm. Englewood Cliffs, NJ: Prentice-Hall.

Etzioni A (1961) A Comparative Analysis of Complex Organisations. Power, Involvement and their Correlates. New York: Free Press of Glencoe. Compare with the revised analysis in Etzioni A (1995) The Spirit of Community. New York: Harper Collins.

Fritchie R (1997) Personal communication. This sentence is borrowed from the (unpublished) speeches of Dame Renee Fritchie, Chair, South and West Regional Health Authority, 1995–97. See, for example, her foreword in Key P et al (1997) The Unsupported Middle. Oxford: Radcliffe Medical Press.

Ham C (1992) Health Policy in Britain, 3rd Edn. London: Macmillan.

Holden J, Spooner A (1997) Choosing between major quality assurance schemes for general practice. Primary Care, FT Healthcare 7(8): 7–10.

Irvine D, Irvine S (1996) The Practice of Quality. Oxford: Radcliffe Medical Press.

McKeon A J (1996) Making it happen. In Meads G (Ed.) A Primary Care-led NHS: Putting it into Practice. London: Churchill Livingstone.

Meads G (Ed.) (1995) Future Options for General Practice. Oxford: Radcliffe Medical Press.

Meads G (1996) Future options for general practice. British Journal of Health Care Management 2(7): 372–4.

Meads G. (1997). Power and Influence in the NHS: Oceans without Continents. Oxford: Radcliffe Medical Press.

Muir Gray J (1997) Evidence-based Healthcare. London: Churchill Livingstone.

National Health Service Executive (1994) Developing NHS Purchasing and General Practice Fundholding: Towards a Primary-care Led NHS. EL(94)79. London: NHSE.

National Health Service Executive (1995) Priorites and Planning Guidance for the NHS 1996/97. London: NHSE.

National Health Service Executive (1997) Changing the Internal Market. EL(97)33. Leeds: NHSE.

National Primary Care Research and Development Centre (1997) 1996/97 Annual Report. Manchester: NPCRDC.

Pietroni P, Pietroni C (Eds) (1996) Innovation in Community Care and Primary Health. London: Churchill Livingstone.

Plamping D (1995) Exploring New Roles in General Practice. London: King's Fund Primary Care Group (unpublished).

Robinson B (1993) Lyme cordial. Health Service Journal 103: 20–2.

Robinson B (1994) Integrating health and social care: the Lyme Community Care Unit. Community Care Management and Planning 2(5): 139–43.

Secretary of State for Health (1996a) Primary Care: The Future – Choice and Opportunity. London: HMSO.

Secretary of State for Health (1996b) Primary Care: Delivering the Future. London: HMSO.

World Health Organisation (1978) Primary Health Care: Report of the International Conference on Primary Health Care, Alma-Ata, USSR. Geneva: WHO.

Chapter 3
Nursing: responding to the primary care-led NHS

Fiona Ross

Introduction

The aim of this chapter is to explore current and important issues in primary health and community care from the perspective of nursing. The framework of nursing in primary care is changing rapidly. It is anticipated that change will be continuous and to some extent unpredictable. The boundaries between nursing disciplines in the community are shifting as new approaches to primary health care develop. Thus this chapter focuses as far as possible on generic nursing issues in the primary health care setting. It is clear that there are distinct roles in community nursing (district nursing, practice nursing and health visiting), but as a group they face shared and common challenges, and in order to understand these, it is helpful to take a common approach.

Definitions

Primary health care nurses are defined in *New World, New Opportunities* (National Health Service Management Executive, 1993) as those nurses working outside hospital who have been fully prepared through training and education for the clinical responsibilities needed to deliver primary health care in the community; these are mainly health visitors, district nurses, school nurses, practice nurses, community psychiatric nurses, community mental handicap nurses, occupational health nurses and a range of specialist nurses (National Health Service Management Executive, 1993). The work therefore embraces nursing care, treatment, investigations, support, health promotion, public health and working for health in communities and in alliance with other organizations.

43

It is not surprising if the profession is confused about what terms to use when there are conflicting messages coming from professional leaders. Government policy uses the term 'primary health care nursing', outlined above, whereas professional policy from the United Kingdom Central Council for Nursing, Midwifery and Health Visiting (UKCC) and the English National Board for nursing and midwifery (ENB) use the term 'community health care nursing, (UKCC, 1994). However, the term 'primary health care nursing' is beginning to gain currency in government reports. This may be because the term fits the policy drive for a primary care-led NHS. Critics may argue that taking this route will mean that nursing will be subsumed by the medical model of primary care, which focuses on cure rather than care, with underpinnings from the biosciences rather than the social sciences. This sort of argument probably does not lead very far. Nursing should be confident enough and believe enough in its distinct role to take part, together with other key players – namely GPs – not only in the delivery of care, but also in initiating, leading and evaluating changes that affect nursing and its client groups.

The policy context of primary care nursing

The year 1996 saw a plethora of policy documents on primary care (e.g. Secretary of State for Health, 1996a, 1996b), the culmination of a government listening exercise and the consultation discussed in Chapter 2. As earlier chapters noted, there have been many changes during the 1990s since the NHS reforms were first mooted: GP fundholding, the Community Care Act, the Health of the Nation strategy, the internal market and the primary care-led NHS. These changes include the introduction of contracting and the separation of purchaser and provider functions, as well as the introduction of a health-driven strategy with its emphasis on interagency partnerships, and professionals working together to meet targets for health. The central tenets of the reforms are that care provided by the health service should be efficient, effective, responsive, health oriented, appropriate to the user and properly evaluated. This means that primary health care nursing is required to focus on:

- quality assurance;
- accessibility to services and practitioners;
- assessment, care management and developing tailored care plans;
- working collaboratively with other professionals, patients and their carers to ensure continuity;

- safe, effective, evidence-based clinical practice;
- pre-eminently involving the user centre stage.

Reorganizations and a fair chunk of optimistic policy rhetoric have served to change the shape of nursing in primary care. In whatever ways the new Labour government shapes its health policy, 1996 was important because, for the first time, policy documents reflected what seems to be an emerging acceptance that primary care is not synonymous with general practice. Indeed, there was confirmation that it is made up of many professional voices and that many of the key players are nurses (the term being used generically here) as well as GPs.

Therefore the major themes of this chapter are drawn from issues highlighted in the 1996 White Papers (which have been subsequently reflected in the 1997 White Paper) and discussed from the perspective of nursing in primary care. These include nursing workload, the development of new roles and organizational models, the assessment of health needs, care management and health checks for people over 75 years of age, the shifting balance of care, the meaning of caring in the context of the internal market and evaluation. This chapter is written from the perspective of the author's background in district nursing and social policy and it highlights key issues for nursing in contemporary primary care. No claims are made for comprehensiveness because of the constraints of space.

Fairness and equitable distribution of the nursing resource

'Total spending on primary care (including community health services) is around £12.45 billion. This represents over 36% of total NHS spending. If primary care is to continue to make a growing contribution to health care it needs to get a fair share of overall NHS resources' (Secretary of State for Health, 1996b). The White Paper *Primary Care: Delivering the Future* highlighted three important issues:

1. a fairer distribution of resources across the country;
2. a more appropriate balance of resources between primary and secondary care;
3. greater flexibility in the use of resources locally.

There are clearly many complex issues involved in the discussion of the distribution of health services across the primary and secondary care divide. Health authorities facing financial pressure are having to make decisions about disinvestment from community health services to redirect resources to prop up struggling acute services (Godfrey and Cassidy, 1996). Media and political attention is easily drawn to the closure of hospital wards, but cutting numbers of community nurses and closing a community clinic usually passes quietly, noticed by few.

It is clear that the shift in balance of care means that nurses in the community are experiencing increased workload pressures from:

- the impact of an ageing population;
- people discharged from hospital 'sicker and quicker';
- acute care at home, for example renal dialysis;
- increased palliative and terminal care at home, for example for HIV/AIDS;
- community care and packages of home care;
- more demands from training and clinical supervision.

In the light of these pressures, it is interesting to look at the staffing figures of nurses in the community. In 1994, 18 413 (whole-time equivalent, WTE) nursing staff were employed in district nursing in England, representing about 40% of all primary health care nurses (Department of Health, 1996). There has been a decline in the number of qualified district nurses of 16.4% and a fall in that of health visitors by 10.1% since 1990. The fall in number in district nursing has resulted in a more dilute grade mix in which less than half of those over 18 000 WTEs in 1994 (47%) have a district nursing qualification (Audit Commission, 1997). Even with grade mix and the increasing use of D and F grades in district nursing, this does not compensate for the overall decrease. As well as these overall trends in workforce statistics, the number of places for district nursing and health visiting training has fallen and the district nursing workforce is ageing (Audit Commission, 1997). These trends are in marked contrast to those in practice nursing, which has seen remarkable growth. Over the past 10 years, numbers have increased more than four-fold (Secretary of State for Health, 1996a). It seems that these simple figures point to where the balance of care is shifting – not to community Trusts but into general practice. Undoubtedly, there is an enormous job to be done within the general practice setting for practice nurses, particularly in the field of chronic disease management, which is moving increasingly from secondary care to primary care. Practice nurses therefore play an increasingly important role in running health promotion clinics, in the management of minor illness and in providing health counselling. It would not be surprising – and there is some anecdotal evidence – to find that there is a drift of health visiting, district nursing and midwifery expertise into practice nursing as this discipline expands. This redistribution of work, the range of expertise required and the lack of standardized training in practice nursing highlights the need for education to support this developing workforce. At the same time, it is important to recognize the need to support the increasingly pressurized and denuded disciplines of district nursing and health visiting.

New nursing roles in primary health care

The devolution of decision-making and the promotion of services appropriate to the needs of local communities inevitably result in local organizational diversity. The White Paper *Primary Care: Delivering the Future* states that 'as the service develops, the need for improved team-working and partnership will grow' (Secretary of State for Health, 1996b). This has implications for the development of nursing in primary care, particularly in terms of better teamworking within primary health care, developing professional roles, partnerships with health authorities, secondary care and local authorities. These policies, as well as the focus on primary health care as the driving force for change, mean that the roles of nurses in primary health care will change to meet new demands, and new roles will emerge. In the first half of the 1990s, skill mix has been confused with grade mix, and doctor substitution has been debated in relation to nurses' extended roles. There have been arguments on the one hand for a generic worker, whilst on the other, there is the thrust for greater autonomy for nurses, as seen for example in the emerging role of the nurse practitioner and the development of nurse prescribing. Finally, there is tension between the contrasting approaches of individualistic care and public health approaches, highlighted by Meads in Chapter 2.

Skill mix has been defined as the balance of relevant skills and experience required by staff working in a particular environment with a specific client group. This balance will relate to the nature of the experience and educational background of the staff concerned and the nature of the work (Gibbs et al, 1991). However, grade mix is the profile of the mix of grades of staff in a team, which may not reflect the skills of the staff at all. In other words, grade mix is a management tool for assigning grades and rank to staff that may not necessarily be informed by qualifications or competencies. This distinction is important in the following discussion of developments in nursing organization in nursing care.

The self-managed/integrated nursing team

There are many local variations in new primary care organizational development, one of which is the self-managed team (also called independent or integrated nursing team), based in general practice. It usually consist of a team of health visitors, practice nurses and district nurses with a variety of parallel relationships with other members of the primary care team, for example midwives, therapists and GPs. The team may manage the full budget, the staff budget or none at all. They may be charged with developing services or relationships with other disciplines or agencies; they may have the authority to recruit, select and decide on the skill/grade mix of staff. The nature and level of management support to such teams varies (Community and District Nursing Association, 1997).

This development is being driven by the slimming of management structures in community Trusts and the need to respond to questions that purchasers ask about the efficient and optimum skill mix between GPs, nurses and therapists necessary to deliver effective and quality care. Most schemes to date have been local developments with little evaluation. The York work on skill mix diversity and delegation has highlighted the fact that patterns of GP delegation, skill mix and workload vary across primary care teams. There is some evidence that this variation may reflect features of the individual practices' organization and working style (Jenkins-Clarke et al, 1997).

In the Tile Hill project in Coventry (Reid, 1993), Roy's GP-managed model (Roy, 1990) was developed so that the nurses from a variety of disciplines formed and functioned as a nursing provider unit. One of the results of this experiment was that changes in use of skill came about through nurse participation rather than as a result of top-down management decisions. A second model in Essex Rivers Healthcare (Edwards, 1994) set up a multi-agency steering group and seconded a health visitor to provide nursing advice to nursing teams in four GP practices. The aims of this project were to provide an efficient nursing service for the practice population whilst ensuring expertise and avoiding duplication. It is hoped that nurses will be able to question and challenge the traditional boundaries between their roles and improve the integration and continuity of care. Premier Health has also piloted a model of organizing nursing with the aims of increasing co-operation and flexibility, reducing professional boundaries and improving teamwork among nurses working in the primary health care team (Morgan, 1994). This means that GP-employed and attached nursing staff work together to plan, prioritize, implement and evaluate their work to maximize the contribution to nursing care. To do this, one member of the team assumes the role of leader to facilitate team and role development. This role is rotated and is considered to be enabling and non-hierarchical. The focus of this work starts with a practice population profile (described below) and assumes autonomy as well as financial control for the nursing team.

The focus of this author's recent work with colleagues was the assessment of the change in use of skills before and 1 year after the introduction of a nurse-managed team in a first wave GP fundholding practice (the manager in this case being a district nurse). Although at the start of the study it was planned to use the measures of workload and activity only with the nurses, the GPs also volunteered to take part. Self-completion time diaries and case record forms were used to note the use of time and skill across a range of activities, including treatment, investigation, assessment, health promotion/advice and administration. This quantitative data was fed back to nurse participants in semi-structured interviews to elicit their views on the activity and workload data. The results showed that there was a 17% increase in the number of patients seen by the practice nurses, district nurses and health visitors at the end of the year, and that, overall, more assessments, treatment advice sessions and investigations were carried out by the time of the second audit. The views reported by the nurses and GPs at the second audit showed a questioning and evaluative approach to the changing organization and to nursing roles and skills (Rink et al, 1996). The development of this method has been reported (Godfrey et al, 1997) and is being used in further work with a variety of integrated nursing team models in place in three health authorities.

Substitution or extended roles?

The boundaries between nursing and medicine are shifting. The factors influencing this include projected falls in the GP workforce following declining recruitment to the speciality, increased retirement rates and a shift towards part-time working favoured by the increasing proportion of women in medicine (General Medical Services Committee, 1996). This decline in the workforce means that levels of care delivery cannot be sustained and the increased demands for care cannot be met unless there is some redistribution of work. The substitution of nurses undertaking medical tasks is one solution to this problem. The issue of substitution inevitably raises some interesting issues for nurses in primary care. It is reasonably straightforward to conceptualize the substitution of medical tasks by practice nurses doing them, because their work is largely defined by the needs of the practice, and the GP is their manager and employer. Indeed, the development of practice nurses' work and the emergence of the nurse practitioner in the general practice setting is evidence of this.

Substitution assumes, in this case, that a clinical service (traditionally carried out by doctors) is delegated to and managed by another professional group. This notion does not fit easily with some aspects of the health visiting and district nursing role, particularly in relation to services for which there is little other provision, for example in deprived inner city areas and work with marginalized client groups such as the homeless (Atkinson, 1987). This is especially the case in health visiting, in which the public health role has been population rather than practice based. For example, in inner city areas where GP services are often underdeveloped, the provision of child health and community services provides an invaluable contribution and fills the gap left by inadequate GP services. Therefore substitution cannot be applied in a blanket fashion to primary care nurses, for whom the priorities of care, history, professional identity, funding base, scope of clinical decision-making and management relationships are different and may be in conflict with the values and priorities of the GP. Thus the analysis of manpower needs in primary care must take account of the context and roles of the key players as well as the tensions around professional boundaries.

Nurse specialists in primary care

As a result of the changing balance of care from the secondary to primary care sector, there has been an increase in the development of specialist and outreach nurses who are often part of the secondary care power base. The jury is still out on specialist practice in nursing. Although the notion of the advanced practitioner has been dropped, there is still considerable confusion over educational level, role expectations and the standing of new roles such as that of the nurse practitioner, discussed below. While the UKCC and the profession debates the issue, the service is rapidly developing specialist roles, but without the coherent educational strategy to underpin the developments. The nurse specialist in primary care has tended to develop in areas of chronic/continuing care, for example continence, palliative care and rehabilitation, that have been marginalized and poorly served by generalists. Issues of control and tension between the specialist and generalist roles have emerged in the literature. Haste and MacDonald (1992) found that specialist nurses were valued as a resource by generalist nurses (district nurses), but other work has identified that the generalist district nurse perceives the threat of role erosion (Griffiths, 1994).

Nurse practitioners

Some would say that there have always been nurse practitioners in primary health care, for example the triple-duty nurse working as a health visitor, district nurse and midwife. These posts still exist today in parts of the UK, especially in remote, sparsely populated rural communities such as the Western Isles of Scotland. There are also nurses practising independently and autonomously in a range of specialities such as midwifery and occupational health.

The nurse practitioner concept originated in the USA in the 1960s in rural or inner city primary care where the recruitment of doctors was difficult. Further training was given (now in the form of a 2-year Masters course) enabling nurses to assess and manage patient care problems that would normally have been dealt with by family doctors. The definition of the nurse practitioner role includes:

- assessment, including physical examination and history-taking;
- the management of illness and continuity of care;
- health promotion and support;
- collaboration with physicians and other health workers to provide co-ordinated care.

The nurse practitioner role shares some of the characteristics of that of the specialist nurse in that there is an advanced knowledge base, but the primary distinction is that there is direct patient access. There is also an element of independent decision-making guided by protocols and usually taking place within the team. Nurse practitioners are trained to make diagnoses and treat at least the simpler and common conditions.

A review of the American and British literature indicates that, during the 1970s and early 80s, there was considerable debate and research on the role of the nurse practitioner in the USA. These studies focused on acceptability to patients/physicians, the work environment, health outcomes and cost.

Although old, one of the best known studies is the Burlington randomized controlled trial (Spitzer et al, 1974). The initiative to develop a nurse practitioner service came from over-burdened family doctors in primary care. They trained nurses in clinical decision-making for common presenting problems in primary care. The evaluation consisted of the random allocation of patients to a nurse practitioner or a doctor for any first contact. Out of a total of 392 episodes of care, nurse management was rated as adequate in 69% of cases compared with 66% of cases in the doctor group. Nurse practitioners were able to function independently in 67% of the patient contacts, and the vast majority of patients (96%) were satisfied on seeing the nurse. This study can be criticized in that it was carried out in one practice with a small number of nurses and doctors, and there was clearly some vested interest in its success because the investigators were also the participating medical practitioners. However, it is a rare example of an evaluation of a new role using the experimental method.

In Britain until recently, evaluation studies focused on small-scale or single nurse practitioner innovations. There is recent work systematically evaluating the nurse practitioner role in acute (Dowling et al, 1995) and accident and emergency settings (Tye, 1997). However, Stillwell's work in Birmingham is the best-known primary care example. Her research suggested that the focus of the nurse practitioner's work in general practice is the holistic care of the client. Assessment and treatment are broader based than with the doctor and include concerns with rehabilitation, coping and the psychosocial aspects of illness (Stillwell et al, 1987).

South East Thames RHA evaluated 20 nurse practitioners working in a range of settings including open-access community settings, accident and emergency departments and primary care alongside GPs (Touche Ross, 1994). On all sites, the evaluation showed high levels of patient satisfaction with the nurse practitioners. In primary care, the nurse practitioners were found to provide a safe, valued and beneficial service to selected groups of patients. However, it was not clear to what extent this service could be provided equally well by a health visitor or district nurse with an extended role; thus more careful evaluation is needed.

Despite the work by Stillwell, the nurse practitioner role is still contested within the profession, some arguing that medical substitution will diminish the focus of nursing to a biomedical, mechanistic approach, thus subjugating the importance of care to the imperative of cure.

Nurse prescribing

The Cumberlege report (Department of Health and Social Security, 1986) recommended that 'suitably qualified' community nurses should, as part of their everyday nursing practice, be able to prescribe from a limited list of items. Three groups of patients were highlighted as being most likely to benefit from nurse prescribing. These were patients with post-operative wounds, patients with stomas or catheters and groups such as homeless families who may not be registered with a GP. Despite the relatively quick introduction of the prescribing legislation, the implementation of this policy has been fermenting slowly for 10 years while pilot sites have been evaluated (Luker et al, 1997). There have been areas of nursing practice, for example triple-duty nursing, occupational health nursing and family planning, in which prescribing decisions have long been in existence, but nurse prescribing is a way of legitimizing this. There is an interesting argument around whether this is an aspect of substitution, the development of nursing autonomy or an example of how professions renegotiate boundaries in a health care system permanently in flux (Shepherd et al, 1996). The pre- and post-registration training implications for the community nursing workforce are considerable and should include therapeutics, advanced communication with other professionals and practical aspects of dispensing.

Assessment in primary care

Assessment in primary and community care has become a key priority in policy and practice over the past 7 years. In order to purchase appropriate health care for their resident populations, commissioning agencies need to profile or describe the characteristics of their populations. A brief discussion of some of the issues in health profiles in community care follows. GPs, health visitors and nurses are expected to make use of the population profiles carried out by their public health department. Sometimes, they carry out this work themselves. This raises many problems, because the arena of health needs assessment is as yet an inexact science with many methodological problems. Furthermore, it highlights one of the vital and important challenges for nurses in primary care, whatever their discipline, which is the twin requirements to assess and give care to individuals within the context of assessing and understanding the wider needs of population groups within the community. These demands raise some very difficult questions about the interface of individual practitioners with a wider public health role. In assessment, epidemiological data will be drawn from a number of sources, including census, population morbidity data and the use of services (Victor, 1996). In addition, detailed knowledge held by nurses and especially health visitors is important in practice profiles. Disentangling the differences between an individual and a community approach is important. This is beginning to happen in some circumstances: district nurses are taking on the challenges of community-based assessments and acknowledging the importance of taking initiatives in health promotion rather than making referrals to others (Ross and Elliott, 1995), and health visitors are redefining their role and establishing their focus of practice to public health (Cowley, 1997).

Assessment and care management in community care

Despite the rhetoric of health profiling, the real emphasis in the NHS and community care reforms is on individual assessment. This is driven by a funding mechanism that uses assessment as a means of defining costs through the packages of care identified for each individual. Therefore the key objectives are to establish priorities, allocate resources, describe case mix and plan individual care. Assessment is discussed in relation to the screening of people aged 75 years and over in general practice, as well as to care management and the interface of primary and secondary care.

The community care changes gave responsibility to local authorities for the finance of all publicly supported long-term care outside the NHS (Department of Health, 1989a). Social security funding under income support arrangements was run down and reallocated through the revenue support grant to local authorities. The majority of this reallocation was to purchase packages of care from the independent sector. The operationalization of community care in local authorities has affected nursing in a variety of ways, but most importantly it has highlighted the difficulties of working with an arbitrary separation between health and social care. There are many examples of this, but the issue of bathing raises most controversy. Bathing was a service that, in the past, was carried out by auxiliaries in district nursing teams. Now this service has been passed over to social services unless there is a medical need. The effect of this is that bathing is no longer available as hard-pressed social service departments are only able to provide social baths to those eligible clients, which is usually only those with severe dependency needs (Victor, 1997).

Theoretically, care management may be carried out by any appropriately qualified professional from the health or social sector (Department of Health, 1989b). In practice, this has not happened, because the concept was inadequately defined and the process not sufficiently thought through in terms of the link between assessment, purchasing and resource allocation. Bergen (1994) surveyed 98 health authorities to identify what she defined as case management-related activities among community nurses. It is not surprising that the findings showed a variety of roles reported as care management, but the most frequent role was carried out by community psychiatric nurses, and purchasing of services only featured in 13% of cases, in contrast to assessment, which was undertaken in 97.5% of cases. There are reported cases of district nurses carrying out joint assessments using a core assessment tool (Korczak, 1993; Ross and Tissier, 1997).

Assessment and the over-75 years in general practice

The 1990 GP Contract made it a requirement for GPs to carry out an annual assessment of their registered patient population over 75 years of age. The focus of the assessment is on social needs, mobility, mental health, sensory needs, continence, functional performance and medication. There have been reservations about the cost-effectiveness of universal 'screening' versus the targeted assessment of people in at-risk groups (Illife et al, 1991). In a national survey carried out by Chew et al (1994), it was found that a variety of methods of assessment were in use in general practice, varying from opportunistic doctor-led assessment during a consultation to a practice nurse-led recall and assessment, and, less frequently, assessments carried out by practice-attached health visitors or district nurses. Furthermore, it was found that a variety of checklists or interview schedules had been adopted.

An important question is who in the health care team is most appropriate to carry out the assessment. There appears from the literature to be some ambivalence. In one study, the majority of primary care team members thought that the health visitor was the most appropriate health professional, although half the health visitors themselves disagreed, seeing their priorities as being with the 0–5-year-olds (Tremellen and Jones, 1989). Most studies have, in fact, identified the practice nurse as doing the majority of the assessments (Brown et al, 1992; Tremellen, 1992), with doctors doing some, rare inputs from health visitors and district nurses and, in some cases, assessments being carried out by volunteers (Carpenter and Demopoulos, 1990).

The meaning of caring in a market culture

The internal, or quasi-market as some commentators are now describing it, has led to a radical change to the way in which care is defined. Care has become a marketable commodity, and professionals are implicitly part of market transactions. This is particularly marked at the social care boundary with health care, for example the provision of the 'social bath' or aids and equipment, which are means tested. Thus the market approach to health care has challenged some fundamental values and beliefs of many working in the health service. Some have difficulty in reconciling the concepts of efficiency and value for money with the 'special experience of caring' from which they draw meaning and job satisfaction.

Traynor (1995) highlights the uncertainty and declining morale and job satisfaction among community nurses and contrasts this with the relative job satisfaction of practice nurses. This may be linked to the manpower trends discussed earlier and the associated enhanced resourcing and infrastructure of general practice compared with community Trusts.

This low morale in nursing is mirrored in general practice. Patrick Pietroni (1996), in his inaugural lecture at the University of Westminster, entitled 'A primary care-led NHS: trick or treat?', describes the mid-life crisis of general practice – the despair of losing what one once possessed; the fatigue associated with realizing that the task is beyond our capacities; the anger associated with feeling that no one really understands; and the spiritual ennui and confusion linked to loss of direction.

These feelings are probably common across the primary care team. Although the influencing factors may be different, the end result is more or less the same. In health visiting, the public health role is seen by many to be challenged by the practice organization of general practice and the different priorities of care. District nurses, as mentioned earlier, are also experiencing a massive change in their workloads and job orientation.

Developing professional knowledge

The final part of this chapter is a discussion of the development of professional knowledge in order to build and strengthen primary care. What does developing an evidence-based service mean in primary care, and what form should education take to prepare practitioners for a new kind of service?

Measuring outcomes is not the prerogative of one professional group, nor should it rely on one type of method or one sort of evidence. Providers need to know what constitutes good care and how it can best be delivered so that it can be repeated or amended. The purchaser will need information for an overview of the balance of care provision to meet user needs. The primary care team may need to decide whether the task is to evaluate the service as a whole, including patient satisfaction, or to measure changes in health behaviour or status.

There is a hierarchy of types of evidence that are given greater or lesser value in health care evaluation. Quantitative data, particularly produced by the randomized control trial, are given considerable credence in supporting and justifying decisions on which to base practice. In contrast, qualitative data are often seen as soft and limited, because of their lack of generalizability. Kendall (1997) challenges the notion that the only respectable and credible evidence for professional decision-making comes from the clinical trial approach. 'To limit our evidence to the RCT (randomized controlled trial) as providing the best evidence, denies the rich diversity of human experience which nurses working in the community have the privilege to be intimate with' (Kendall, 1997).

Preparing nurses to work with greater autonomy and with new skills informed by research evidence in an arena where the parameters of practice are changing is vital but complex. It needs to take place at a number of levels: pre-registration and post-registration with a multi-disciplinary component throughout. Nurses in primary care need more input on epidemiology, health promotion, communication skills, policy and ethical dilemmas, and ways of responding with new clinical skills to complex and increasingly acute problems in the community. In addition, nurses need to develop and be supported in a continuous way with critical appraisal skills to make sense of and use appropriately research literature in primary care.

As well as moving towards professional decision-making informed by evidence, there is a need for education to fit the purpose of tomorrow's health service and to prepare and support an appropriate skill mix of practitioners to meet the health needs of the 21st century. The service will need flexible practitioners capable of innovation, collaboration and sustaining change.

The policy imperative identified unequivocally in *Primary Care: Delivering the Future* (Secretary of State for Health, 1996b) is the need to have a collaborative approach to delivery supported by more multi-disciplinary training. At a pre-qualifying level, there is evidence of shared learning between nursing and professionals allied to medicine, but there is little involvement of medical students (Centre for the Advancement of Interprofessional Education, 1996). Again, in continuing education, one of the difficulties seems to be finding examples of courses that have a multi-disciplinary group including doctors (Storrie, 1992). There are many reasons for this gap between the rhetoric and the practice, perhaps one of the most fundamental being the existence of different stakeholders and funding streams for education, both pre- and post-qualifying, for health care professionals. Although there are some encouraging signs that the funding of practice nurse education is becoming integrated with the NHS consortia of purchasing Trusts, there are still issues about funding for locum cover to release staff for training.

Conclusion

The shape of services in primary care is changing rapidly and unpredictably, and nurses need the skills to respond appropriately. Whilst there is evidence of low morale, there are also examples of initiatives that provide opportunities for developing quality nursing care in the community. Primary care nurses need to find a shared future that is health focused and evidence based but does not forget the need to provide continuous and family-centred care.

References

Atkinson J (1987) 'I just exist': Glasgow's single homeless men. Community Outlook (November): 12–15.
Audit Commission (1997) 'Wards without Walls': A Study of the Efficiency

and Effectiveness of Community Nursing Services. Consultative document. London: Audit Commission.

Bergen A (1994) Case management in the community: identifying a role for nursing. Journal of Clinical Nursing Care 3(4): 251–7.

Brown K, Williams E, Groom L (1992) Health checks on patients 75 years and over in Nottinghamshire after the new contract. British Medical Journal 305: 619–21.

Carpenter G, Demopoulos G (1990) Screening elderly people in the community: controlled trial of dependency surveillance using a questionnaire administered by volunteers. British Medical Journal 300: 1253–6.

Centre for the Advancement of Interprofessional Education (1996) Developing Shared Learning between Medical and Nursing Students. London: CAIPE.

Chew C, Wilkin D, Glendinning C (1994) Annual assessment of patients aged 75 years and over: general practitioners' and practice nurses' views and experiences. British Journal of General Practice 44: 263–7.

Community and District Nursing Association (1997) Position Statement on Self-managed Teams. London: CDNA.

Cowley S (1997) Public health values in practice: the case of health visiting. Critical Public Health 7: 83–97.

Department of Health (1989a) Caring for People. London: HMSO.

Department of Health (1989b) Working for Patients. Cmnd 55. London: HMSO.

Department of Health (1996) Health and Personal Social Services Statistics 1996. London: Stationery Office.

Department of Health and Social Security (1986) Neighbourhood Nursing: A Focus for Care. (Chairman: Julia Cumberlege). London: HMSO.

Dowling S, Barrett S, West R (1995) With nurse practitioners, who needs house officers? British Medical Journal 311: 309–13.

Edwards M (1994) Self managed teams. Presentation at the NHSME Primary Health Care Seminar 'Into the future: beyond audit to quality', London.

General Medical Services Committee (1996) Medical Workforce Task Group report. London: British Medical Association.

Gibbs I, McCaughan D, Griffiths M (1991) Skill mix in nursing: a selective review of the literature. Journal of Advanced Nursing 16: 242–9.

Godfrey K, Cassidy J (1996) Axe hangs over community care. Nursing Times 92: 20–5.

Godfrey E, Rink P, Ross F (1997) Measuring the workload of integrated nursing teams in general practice. British Journal of Community Health Nursing 2(7): 350–5.

Griffiths J (1994) Community nurse attitudes to the clinical specialist. Nursing Times 90: 39–42.

Haste F, MacDonald L (1992) Evaluating the impact of a clinical nurse specialist in community nursing: perceptions of specialist to district nurse. International Journal of Nursing Studies 29(1): 37–47.

Illife S, Haines A, Gallivan S, Booroff A, Goldenberg E, Morgan P (1991) Assessment of elderly people in general practice: social circumstances and mental status. British Journal of General Practice 41: 9–12.

Jenkins-Clarke S, Carr-Hill R, Dixon P, Pringle M (1997) Skill Mix in Primary Care: A Study of the Interface between the General Practitioner and other Members of the Primary Health Care Team. York: University of York, Centre for Health Economics.

Kendall S (1997) What do we mean by evidence?: implications for primary health care nursing. Journal of Interprofessional Care II(I): 23–34.

Korczak E (1993) Joint assessment. Primary Health Care 3(2): 8–10.

Luker K, Austin L, Hogg C, Willcock J (1997) Evaluation of nurse prescribing. York: University of York.

Morgan M (1994) Using teamwork to increase quality. Presentation at the NHSME Primary Health Care Seminar 'Into the future: beyond audit to quality', London.

National Health Service Management Executive (1993) New World, New Opportunities. London: HMSO.

Pietroni P (1996) A primary care-led NHS: trick or treat? Lecture given at the University of Westminster, London.

Reid T (1993) Joint input. Nursing Times 89(47): 30–2.

Rink P, Ross F, Godfrey E, Roberts G (1996) The changing use of nursing skills in general practice. British Journal of Community Nursing 1(6): 363–9.

Ross F, Elliott M (1995) Innovations in Community Nursing. Edinburgh: Community and District Nursing Association.

Ross F, Tissier J (1997) The care management interface with general practice: a case study. Health and Social Care in the Community 5(3): 153–61.

Roy S (Chairman) (1990) Report of the Working Group, Nursing in the Community. London: HMSO.

Secretary of State for Health (1996a) Primary Care: The Future – Choice and Opportunity. London: HMSO.

Secretary of State for Health (1996b) Primary Care: Delivering the Future. London: HMSO.

Shepherd E, Rafferty A M, James V (1996) Prescribing the boundaries of nursing practice: professional regulations and nurse prescribing. Nursing Times (Research) 1(6): 465–78.

Spitzer W, Sackett D, Sibley J (1974) The Burlington randomised trial of the nurse practitioner. New England Journal of Medicine 290(5): 251–6.

Stillwell B, Greenfield S, Drury V, Hull F (1987) A nurse practitioner in general practice: working styles and patterns of consultation. Journal of the Royal College of General Practice 37: 154–7.

Storrie J (1992) Mastering interprofessionalism – an enquiry into the development of Masters programmes with an interprofessional focus. Journal of Interprofessional Care 6(3): 253–61.

Touche Ross (1994) Evaluation of Nurse Practitioner Pilot Projects. Summary Report. Surrey: National Health Service Management Executive/South Thames.

Traynor M (1995) Job satisfaction and morale of nurses in NHS Trusts. Nursing Times 91(26): 42–5.

Tremellen J (1992) Assessment of patients aged over 75 years in general practice. British Medical Journal 305: 621–4.

Tremellen J, Jones D (1989) Attitudes and practices of the primary health care team towards assessing the very elderly. Journal of the Royal College of General Practitioners 39: 142–4.

Tye C (1997) The emergency nurse practitioner role in major accident and emergency departments: professional issues and the research agenda. Journal of Advanced Nursing 26: 364–70

UKCC (1994) The Future of Professional Practice – the Council's Standards for Education and Practice Following Registration. London: UKCC.

Victor C (1996) Health-needs profiling. In Ross F, Mackenzie A (Eds) Nursing in Primary Health Care. London: Routledge.

Victor C (1997) Community Care and Older People. Cheltenham: Stanley Thornes.

Chapter 4
Promoting interprofessional collaboration: the multi-disciplinary face of primary health care

Pauline Pearson

Introduction

Primary health care – health care that is directly accessible to the public and that seeks to promote their well-being and meet their physical, social and psychological health needs – is a complex activity. Just as the needs of any community are multiple, so also the people and structures that come together to meet those needs are many and various. The WHO (World Health Organisation, 1978) defined primary health care as:

- essential health care;
- the first level of contact;
- practice based on scientifically sound and socially acceptable methods;
- universally accessible;
- involving full participation;
- at a cost that the community and country can afford to maintain.

It went on to indicate that it should reflect the economic and socio-cultural characteristics of the country and address its main health problems in a research-based way, providing 'promotive, preventive, curative and rehabilitative services'. Finally, it indicated that primary health care should involve, 'in addition to the health sector, all related sectors and aspects of national and community development' and that it required 'maximum community and individual self reliance and participation in its planning, operation and control'.

For primary health care in the UK, this means that its aims and objectives must be about both promoting and maintaining health, and doing this collaboratively. Many relevant health risks have been identified for concerted action. The Health of the Nation report (Secretary of State for Health, 1992) highlights, for example, cancers, heart disease, sexually transmitted disease and mental illness. The 1990 General Practice contract recognizes the impact of chronic diseases such as diabetes and asthma (Department of Health and the Welsh Office, 1989).

The Alma-Ata Declaration (World Health Organisation, 1978) makes clear that primary health care should be accessible to everyone, including marginalized groups such as homeless people, people with special needs and people from ethnic minorities. It should be free at the point of care. It is, by definition, the first line of health care. Hence primary care practitioners should be able to offer all the appropriate skills to meet basic needs, and be able to work with a wide range of individuals and agencies beyond health care (e.g. schools, local authorities and industry) to promote overall well-being. They should be both effective in achieving those ends and efficient in doing so, making the optimum use of the available resources. Above all, the Declaration indicates that primary health care should be participative and empowering to the people and communities it serves, offering them respect and shared decision-making rather than seeking to control them. Professionals should be operating collaboratively with communities as well as with each other.

In the UK at present, a significant amount of work formerly undertaken in the 'acute' sector is being undertaken by primary care staff. Hospital-at-home schemes, early discharge programmes and not-so-minor day surgery are just three examples. Primary care staff need to develop new skills in order to facilitate this shift, to work with new clients and new colleagues. Clients should benefit most if these developments rest within the holistic and empowering primary health care approach identified by the WHO. If, instead, the shift is seen primarily as a way of off-loading institutional costs and attitudes into the community, quality will deteriorate. Above all, it will be important to resist a movement towards the 'high tech is more important' view prevalent in hospitals, since it denies the importance of good-quality basic care and health promotion.

Two patterns of working seem likely to become more common. First, primary care staff will have expertise in assessment and initial treatment in a range of areas (see below) and should be able to draw in and integrate more specialist services as necessary. For example, in looking at the needs of a teenager diagnosed with diabetes, they will not only ensure links to local specialist groups, but also make connections to education staff and consider family impact and voluntary agency support. They will filter out services that are inappropriate to an individual's needs. The approach taken may be similar to care management in social services, in which one worker, usually a social worker, is responsible for co-ordinating all the relevant services – from voluntary agencies, from social services and health care – to meet each individual's assessed needs. As noted by Ross (Chapter 3), nurses could play a full part in this, including the management of budgets. Second, as public health becomes a higher priority (Jowell, 1997; Department of Health, 1998), approaches to practice based on the principles of public health and community development will become more common. Practitioners in these roles will be seen as being central to decision-making in the area of service provision. They will have a high level of skill not only in their work with clients, but also in the analysis of local health needs and decision-making concerning how these should be tackled, feeding into locality-based primary care groups.

Areas in which primary care staff are developing expert skills include:

- Health promotion, especially primary prevention, community development and local public health work. Health visitors and other groups, such as school nurses and occupational health staff, currently have the skills required. This work involves wide networks of other colleagues.
- Chronic disease management. Primary care should increasingly be the main provider of, for example, asthma, diabetes and arthritis care. GPs, pharmacists, practice nurses and specialist nurses in primary care are assuming much of the day-to-day support and monitoring of these patients but will liaise with hospital staff, social workers and others on a regular basis.
- The care of older people. Primary care staff are increasingly co-ordinating and providing 'seamless care' to older people with substantial health and social needs, in collaboration with social services and voluntary agencies. They will also need to draw on a wide range of local expert resources.

- ' The care of people with long-term mental illness, especially people with anxiety and depression. Changes in the role of community psychiatric nurses are placing additional pressure on GPs and other team members such as practice nurses and health visitors. This is an area in which new roles might develop to fill the gap.
- The sifting and management of self-limiting and minor health problems, together with the identification and referral of serious health problems. This area of practice is probably one of the most rapidly expanding, with some GPs now working in accident and emergency departments and many more nurse practitioners and specialist nurses seeing patients in minor injury centres (Glasman, 1993) and in out-of-hours centres.
- Provision to marginalized communities or groups, especially those for whom traditional care is not accessible. There is considerable potential for the development of new roles with marginal groups, including finding effective ways of bringing them into decision-making.

To undertake the developing primary care task requires not only GPs, health visitors, district and practice nurses, but also physiotherapists, pharmacists, social workers, speech therapists, chiropodists, dietitians and many more. Each will build on a different foundation in understanding and carrying out his own role and function. It is clearly important to appreciate some of the ways in which these understandings can contrast with or complement each other.

This chapter will seek first to discuss some of the policy shifts that are increasingly encouraging interprofessional collaboration, and second, to outline some of the situations and ways in which collaboration occurs in primary health care. Third, it will discuss some models and theories of collaboration, and ways in which these may need to alter in a changing health care context. It will explore interprofessional collaboration in a complex system – the discharge of patients from hospital – and develop some key areas for exploration in practice. Finally, a brief overview of interprofessional education will be provided.

Interprofessional collaboration: the policy

'Teamwork' in primary care has been government rhetoric since at least 1974, when the then Chief Medical Officer wrote in his Annual Report of the advantages of bringing together doctors and nurses in a multi-disciplinary team (Department of Health and Social Security, 1974). He was writing at a time when district nursing and health visiting were just moving from local authorities into the NHS and there was optimism for a revitalized NHS. At intervals since, governments and professional organizations have continued to extol the virtues of teamwork in primary care (Royal College of Nursing, 1980; Standing Medical Advisory Committee and Standing Nursing and Midwifery Advisory Committee, 1981).

Over recent years, there have been significant changes in the direction of the NHS, with important shifts in the focus of primary health care services. The NHS and Community Care Act changed the structure of the NHS, separating the providers of services from those responsible for identifying population needs, and creating a new approach to the provision of health and social care for a number of disadvantaged and marginal groups. For people with mental health problems, those with physical and complex disabilities and older people, the emphasis of care changed. Provision for continuing care came under the auspices of social services, although with increasing amounts of input from the voluntary and private sectors. Provision in hospitals fell, and much specialist health care work began to move into the community, with new services developing to meet need. Meanwhile, technological change was also leading to reductions in the length of hospital stay, with day surgery, less invasive techniques and the wider availability of effective drugs and portable equipment. The impact of much of this change was that an increasing proportion of patients were dealt with outside traditional acute hospital settings and by a range of agencies and professions.

In 1996, there were three NHS White Papers, two of which culminated in the Primary Care Act of 1997. The first of these, entitled *Primary Care: The Future – Choice and Opportunity* (Secretary of State for Health, 1996a), outlined the structural changes needed in primary health care to produce a more effective service. It formed the core of the Act, allowing for a variation in methods of providing general medical services: not limiting this to doctors, bringing practice nurses within the NHS superannuation scheme and enabling GPs to be employed by other agencies, such as Trusts. It therefore changed many of the relationships within which primary care services were delivered.

The second White Paper, *The National Health Service: A Service with Ambitions* (Secretary of State for Health, 1996b), concerned broader issues. It focused on the need for the NHS to be delivered by a range of knowledgeable practitioners, working together effectively. Its main concerns therefore were to promote effective multidisciplinary working and to develop a knowledgeable and adaptable workforce. Whilst the idea of a 'service with ambitions' disappeared from view with the 1997 change of government, to be replaced eventually at the end of 1997 by the new catch phrase 'modern, dependable' (Secretary of State for Health, 1997a), the content of this White Paper was effectively 'buried but not dead'. A number of areas for development were taken forward by civil servants and found favour in the new administration; in particular, there was recognition of the importance of a long-term strategy for education, to be discussed later in this chapter. This indicates an important shift in focus for professional education and training, and a significant emphasis on interprofessional collaboration.

The third White Paper, *Primary Care: Delivering the Future* (Secretary of State for Health, 1996c), set out six areas for the further development of primary health care. Its key themes included flexibility of approach, knowledge-based decision-making and the increased role of information technology, alongside the need to develop effective professional development and teamworking, and to manage services 'seamlessly' across organizational boundaries. Development funding for a range of pilot projects followed. Projects supported included some examination of locality-based models of commissioning and some exploration of new roles in primary care. Each of these has generated new issues for collaborative working, whether in relation to the context of collaboration or to the roles that collaborate.

Mental health services policy

Since 1990, there has been concern about the shape and delivery of mental health services (see Chapter 6). A number of heavily publicized disasters involving people with severe mental illness (Zito, 1994) led to concerns about the level and quality of 'care' in the community. These concerns culminated in the publication, in 1997, of a Green Paper suggesting a range of organizational models for the management of mental health services (Secretary of State for Health, 1997b). These ranged from a loose collaboration between health and social services, effectively similar to the existing situation and still optional, to the development of a new joint authority for mental health services.

With the subsequent change in government, some of the detail of these options became redundant. However, there were two important messages for primary health care in the mental health Green Paper that did not change significantly. First, it was clear that, once again, policy-makers were struggling with the interface between health and social care, attempting to build a system in which different professionals could collaborate more effectively to deliver patient care. Second, the key client group whose needs were addressed by this Green Paper were people with severe and enduring mental illness, the group who had received the negative publicity noted above. However, research amongst practitioners working in primary health care, especially GPs, highlighted the needs of a far larger group of people with long-term mental health problems: people with problems such as anxiety and depression or schizophrenia, which impair their quality of life, prevent them engaging in significant economic activity and account for a considerable and demanding proportion of a GP's workload (Nazareth et al, 1997; Weich et al, 1997; see also Chapter 6). The Green Paper therefore sent signals to practitioners in primary care that further work will be necessary to highlight the economic and social burden of common health problems, and that the medical model is still strong.

'The New NHS'

At the end of 1997 and the beginning of 1998, there was a further flurry of White and Green Papers and executive letters. For example, Executive Letter EL(97)65 (National Health Service Executive, 1997) invited bids from health authorities and other local agencies to become health action zones. It was envisaged that there would be approximately ten such zones, which would be aimed at reducing inequalities in health, improving services and 'securing better value from the total resources available'. The key mechanism whereby this was to be achieved would be via partnerships between health authorities, local authorities, NHS Trusts, primary care groups, voluntary agencies, private sector providers and higher education. This was to be collaboration at a macro level, targeted towards issues for which there would be significant advantage in breaking down barriers between agencies.

In December 1997, the White Paper concerned with the dismantling of the 'NHS market' was issued (Secretary of State for Health, 1997b). To be 'modern' and 'dependable', the new-style NHS would be 'integrated' and would 'guarantee the highest possible standards of quality and efficiency through the country'. The key changes identified were:

• the development of primary care groups or trusts to bring together GPs and community nurses in order to identify local

health needs and establish, in partnership with other agencies, how best to meet them;
* an emphasis on the more efficient exchange of information within the NHS and with the public;
* the development of central institutes to encourage evidence-based practice and quality improvement.

This White Paper effectively laid the foundations for a more collaborative interagency approach to health needs assessment and provision for the next century.

Finally, in early 1998, a Green Paper on public health was issued (Department of Health, 1998). The main thrust of this was to identify the health targets that would guide the NHS over the next decade. It addressed inequalities in health and health care in relation to children, adults of working age and older people, as well as looking at the overall impact of smoking on health. The key message was the need to look beyond traditional health care into, for example, education, leisure, housing and commerce, and to families and communities as well as individuals, in order to intervene effectively to achieve health.

All of these policy shifts have contributed to a climate that encourages interprofessional collaboration in policy-making, in education and, centrally, in practice, within and beyond the traditional boundaries of primary health care.

Interprofessional collaboration in practice

Professional practice in primary health care involves health promotion, disease prevention, care or cure and rehabilitation. Individual professionals can operate either alone or collaboratively, drawing on the skills and knowledge of colleagues. A range of modes of collaboration can exist.

Relatively few situations in primary care today are addressed by individual professionals without reference to colleagues. Those which are include the management of self-limiting illness by GPs and routine developmental surveillance by health visitors. Many more situations will involve individual professionals in collaboration with each other. Collaboration has been defined as 'working in combination with' (*Concise Oxford Dictionary*, 1990), but also as 'co-operating treacherously with the enemy'. For many members of primary health care teams, collaboration beyond traditional boundaries – perhaps with social services or voluntary agencies in addition to the GP or district nurse – is a somewhat frightening activity akin to the latter, involving, as it does, leaving the relatively cosy certainties of groups one understands well and working instead with people who may be unpredictable because they are not fully understood.

One-to-one collaboration may occur when one primary care professional identifies a need that must be met by another; for example, the GP may identify that a patient needs his ears syringed and refer him on to the practice nurse. The health visitor may highlight that a child has a speech problem and refer him to the speech therapist.

Even more commonly, individual professionals will need to work with a number of others to meet the needs of one or more individual patients. Examples of this sort of collaborative arrangement include a practice-based clinic for patients with asthma or diabetes; in the latter, a GP and a district nurse might work with a chiropodist and a dietitian to meet the needs of people with diabetes on the practice list.

Another example might be the looser working arrangement described by Edward (1997) in relation to the management of care for children with special needs. Unlike the situation in a 'clinic', where professionals meet at one place to collaborate with one or more individuals, professionals in Edward's model relate to one another individually in a range of directions but rarely come together as a group except to plan (for example, at case conferences). More often, she suggests, individual practitioners function with an awareness of the ways in which they can draw on others for support and of the areas where they themselves can offer others help.

At the furthest extreme, collaboration can occur between two or more groups, such as between a team of nursing staff seeking to work together more effectively as an 'integrated team' (see Chapter 3) focusing on, for example, work with older people, and a team of social workers, also trying to work together well and seeking to engage health service staff in useful dialogue about care packages. This example also demonstrates the potential for interagency collaboration that is increasingly part of the wider picture of primary health care painted by the WHO.

The range of models of collaboration described so far is influenced predominantly by the perspective of individual patients. Collaboration beyond that focused on individuals or small groups of patients is relatively rarely described. Community development theory (O'Gorman, 1996) has outlined some of the ways in which communities can be enabled to work with a variety of agencies in order to achieve maximum physical, social and psychological well-being. Some attention was paid, particularly in the early months of the NHS and Community Care Act, to anecdotal accounts of the ways in which Trusts and social services were collaborating in different places (Finlay, 1998; Carlisley, 1993). Other work has described some of the structural levels of collaboration in child health services, for example between school staff, community trust staff, GPs and social services (Smith and Melville, 1996), and in services for older people, in which a very wide range of agencies are drawn together in meeting the needs of frail elderly people (Woodhouse et al, 1997). More complex collaborations can also occur in work with homeless people and in the provision of ambulatory care.

Interprofessional collaboration – theories

The theories that underlie collaboration between practitioners from different professions originate substantially in three main areas. First, there are theories based in sociology and psychology about the working of groups. Second are theories, again mainly from psychology, about communication between individuals. Third come theories derived from management and organizational theory about the working of complex systems, organizations and institutions.

As discussed earlier, collaboration can occur in a one-to-one situation, between individuals in groups and between groups. One of the most widely cited studies of collaboration in primary health care was undertaken in the early 1980s (see Gregson et al, 1991). This research looked in some detail at the characteristics of collaboration in primary care, but did so through the exploration of doctor–nurse pairs. GPs and the district nurses and health visitors aligned or attached to them were interviewed about various aspects of the way in which they operated in relation to each other. The study defined collaboration as 'the exchange of information between individuals involved in the delivery of primary health care, which has the potential for action or joint working in the interests of a common purpose' (Armitage, 1983). Five stages of collaboration were identified, ranging from isolation, through encounter, and then communication, to partial and finally full collaboration. This study found that little collaboration existed in practice. However, it highlighted the importance of the attachment of community nursing staff to a limited number of GPs, a shared day-to-day base, social interaction (for example, the mutual use of first names), commenting on each other's work and an understanding of each other's responsibilities as factors indicating the potential level of collaboration in a setting.

To a large extent these findings are unsurprising if one examines the literature on the psychology of communication. Effective communication requires a range of modes: from formal to informal, from verbal to written. It is facilitated where empathy is displayed and there is a capacity to see things from the other's viewpoint. The development of shared goals, and familiarity with others' roles, facilitates this process. A range of tactics can be employed, intentionally or unintentionally, to influence others; these include ingratiation with people, modelling on 'successful' others and conformity with high status colleagues (Niven, 1994). Being based together facilitates informal as well as formal communication.

Later studies of collaboration in primary care have moved on to look mainly at individuals in groups. For example, West and Poulton (1997a, 1997b) have explored the components of team effectiveness in primary care. Much of the theory underpinning this type of work has been described by them, and others, elsewhere (Poulton and West, 1994). However, some key points are usefully highlighted. Group output is not necessarily greater than the sum of the output of its parts; in fact, Ringelmann's rope-pulling exercise (Ringelmann, 1913) suggests that it could be less. There is evidence that clarity about role and function within a team improves productivity (Weldon and Weingart, 1993). However, the mean productivity of a group may not be as great as the individual productivity of the most able group member.

At this level, effective collaboration depends upon clarity in understanding the different contributions to a whole task and the avoidance of redundant effort. In order to work together effectively, then, individual practitioners need to be able to identify their own contribution to the overall goal and then to articulate it to colleagues and patients. They also need to be able to assert their views in a multidisciplinary setting.

Experimental work by Belbin (1993) has been widely used to determine the individual characteristics of effective team members. Belbin suggested that, at least in achieving a constructed task with a group of people unknown to each other, several types of contribution could be identified. In earlier experimental work, he identified six types (Belbin, 1981); this developed, through reflection on real-life situations, to nine by 1993:

1. *Plant people* are creative problem solvers.
2. *Resource investigators* are extrovert, enthusiastic people who develop contacts.

3. *Co-ordinators* are good at clarifying goals and encouraging deci-
    sion-making, and are also good delegators.
4. *Shapers* thrive on pressure and have the drive to overcome obstacles.
5. *Monitor evaluators* look at all the options and are good at judging.
6. *Teamworkers* are co-operative and diplomatic. They tend to seek
    to avoid friction.
7. *Implementers* turn ideas into practice.
8. *Completers* are conscientious, looking for errors and omissions.
    They deliver on time.
9. *Specialists* contribute knowledge and skills that are relatively rare:
    they are single-minded and dedicated.

However, the roles that people adopt in any team are not readily
distinguishable in day-to-day situations, and are also not mutually
exclusive. Most team members will at some points adopt one role, at
others another. Effective teamwork occurs when the balance of roles
is right.

Øvretveit (1995) builds upon psychological theory to offer an
overview of factors involved in team decision-making and indicates
that effective collaboration builds upon differences within any team,
using these creatively. However, he suggests that where differences
are seen negatively, they become destructive. He divides types of
decision into four:

1. profession-specific decisions, limited to one professional group;
2. care management decisions, which look at decisions in relation to
    co-ordinating services for one client;
3. policy and 'management' decisions, which affect the whole
    'team';
4. planning decisions about client group needs, team objectives and
    plans.

He subsequently looks at ways of making decisions and concludes
that there are five common approaches, ranging from 'practitioner
alone' to 'unanimous'. He suggests that formal decision-making structures can prevent unnecessary conflict and ensure that differences are
worked through appropriately.

Relatively few studies have examined the collaboration between
groups and institutions, that is, at the macro level. Those that have
include an exploratory study of an integrated nursing team in the
context of a wider primary health care team (Black and Hagel, 1995),
which considered the relationship between that team and its 'parent'

primary health care teams, work looking at community development approaches that addresses inter-agency links (Meethan, 1995), and work from McMaster University in Canada (Browne et al, 1996) looking at relationships and outcomes across whole health and social care systems. The theoretical underpinning of work at this level derives from systems theory and work exploring organizational function.

Interprofessional collaboration in 'ordinary' primary health care

Much of what has been written about teamwork in primary care has addressed what is seen as 'ordinary' primary health care. However, it is important in considering this to be aware of two particular areas of debate that influence ideas about teamwork in this context. First, despite the WHO's definition of primary health care, membership of the primary health care team is constructed by different players according to different agendas. Many of those who write about primary health care teams limit their remarks to clinically active team members, thus excluding the crucial contributions of administrative and clerical staff. Others consider the team members paid for by GPs, thus excluding the contributions of staff employed by other organizations, for example staff based in Trusts. Research exploring primary health care team membership (Pearson and van Zwanenberg, 1991) has indicated that core members are identified consistently by a majority of doctors, nurses and administrative staff working in community settings. However, another study looking at team membership in relation to function (Pearson, 1997) indicated that individuals who had themselves been identified by practice managers as primary health care team members did not identify consistent team profiles. Differences in perception related to:

- An awareness of sub-teams. For example, health care assistants and staff nurses were frequently 'invisible', masked by the district nursing sisters in the team.
- The nature of the employment. For example, was this full or part time? One evening receptionist identified a very limited 'team', which reflected the context in which she worked.
- The length of experience/newness. For example, a member of staff who had recently completed an induction programme identified a far broader team membership than similar staff who were

more experienced, or than the same person interviewed after a gap of several months.

Many researchers in the area of primary health care team function deal with these dilemmas by utilizing team membership as defined by individual informants, or groups highlighted as core members (see Øvretveit, 1995, for a discussion of the characteristics of core and peripheral team membership). However, there are some difficulties in this as gate-keepers (the people who enable the researcher to access the team) are often the main arbiters of the sample. Which gate-keeper is selected will thus tend to determine the range of the sample.

Second, although teamwork in primary health care is often viewed as a static phenomenon, to be aspired to and then achieved, the reality appears to be that, as the policy context alters, the players involved in collaboration shift significantly. Usherwood et al (1997) clearly demonstrate some of the alterations in membership of core primary health care teams in Sheffield between 1990 and 1994. Between these years, the greatest shift in team membership occurred following the new GP contract, when large numbers of practice nurses came into post. More recent changes have arisen as a result of the introduction of 'skill mix' into teams, bringing in staff nurses and nursery nurses among others (Brown, 1997). Concerns over coping with mental health have brought counsellors or psychologists into many teams (Young, 1996). Others have been expanded by welfare rights workers (Stacy et al, 1996) and some by nurse practitioners (Stilwell et al, 1987). Yet others have seen the advent of direct access physiotherapy as part of the team (Jones, personal communication, 1998).

Even without contextual change, some changes are likely to occur in the team. Indeed, few work groups will remain stable for more than perhaps a year at a time. It is not therefore appropriate to assume, in promoting interprofessional collaboration, that a one-off intervention will be satisfactory. Promoting and maintaining collaboration will require a longer-term approach, which takes account of changes in team membership as well as changing goals.

'Maintenance' is not generally evaluated. The Health Education Authority (HEA) looked at interprofessional collaboration in primary care in relation to health promotion (Spratley, 1989). Selected members of primary health care teams (two or three per team) were taken on a training session during which they were encouraged to work together effectively and to look at health promotion collaboratively. They were then sent back to try to develop work with their colleagues in the primary health care team. The HEA undertook a limited follow-up 3 months after the original intervention but did not add any further training input. There was no longer-term follow-up of either team function or health promotion activity levels. This study was also limited by the nature of the original intervention, which was restricted to single representatives of key groups (doctors, nurses and administrative staff).

A number of studies have looked at strategies for the promotion of collaborative working within individual practices and primary care teams. Hudson and Bennett (1997), working in Scotland, looked at the impact of a scheme to promote collaborative working in the context of a workforce reporting increasing stress and overload. They used an action research approach to determine the key stressors and facilitate change. They found that practical changes, such as alterations to repeat prescribing systems, were made and maintained. However, they found that methods of feedback to the team needed to be targeted to key groups in order to be effective in facilitating change. Hudson and Bennett also described the impact of the introduction of a post (a patient services manager) to facilitate more effective working in another practice in Tayside, and some of the problems encountered in seeking to change established patterns of working. One of the post-holder's priorities was to improve communication and teamwork within the practice. Meetings were the chief means by which he sought to achieve change. The authors describe the development of successful large-scale strategic meetings but the failure of the group to develop smaller, more focused working groups to move action forward.

Meetings are often regarded as central to 'teamwork' in primary health care. Bennett-Emslie and McIntosh (1995) looked at factors promoting or impeding teamwork in 14 general practices and associated social work teams, and found that their participants identified practice meetings as 'the single most important mechanism for the promotion of teamwork'; such meetings were associated with greater awareness amongst the professionals involved of the range of services available. The authors went on to state that team members themselves believed that opportunities for formal contact of this sort were 'often inadequate'.

Pearson (1997) looked at interprofessional collaboration in two primary health care teams in Newcastle upon Tyne and found that a 1-day 'awayday' could successfully alter participants' perceptions of their place within the team. For example, auxiliaries began by feeling peripheral but ended up feeling that they had a specific contribution to make. Gilley (1996) used a similar questionnaire in Sunderland to determine the level of collaboration in teams where responsibility for nursing management was transferred to the GPs on an experimental basis. She found little or no measurable change on Dyer's scale (Dyer, 1987) in team members' perceptions of their level of collaboration. Interventions of different types have thus produced different results, with causative links being very difficult to determine.

At a more macro level, Thomas and Graver (1997) and Bryar and Bytheway (1996) have described two large-scale approaches to the promotion of interprofessional collaboration in 'ordinary' primary health care. Thomas and Graver worked on the development and evaluation of the Liverpool Primary Health Care Facilitation Project. This utilized a locality-centred approach to the development of more integrated primary health care, seconding staff for sessions each week to contribute to local multi-disciplinary facilitation teams and highlighting a wide range of positive outcomes. Bryar and Bytheway were involved in the Teamcare Valleys initiative in South Wales. This project was funded by the Welsh Office to improve the community health care infrastructure of the area, with particular emphasis on supporting improved teamwork. A multi-disciplinary group undertook a four-pronged programme incorporating education and training, communication, field projects and practical support and advice to facilitate the development of the dispersed and undervalued practices with their attached and aligned staff.

In both of these initiatives, a significant amount of money was required to set up and maintain the project. Although both have apparently been successful in developing more effective collaboration, funding is always more or less finite: Teamcare Valleys was funded for 3 years (1993–96). Both Teamcare Valleys and the Liverpool initiative are, however, projects that involved the development of an approach empowering local practitioners to take their goals forward. It will be important therefore to continue to review the longer-term impact of such large-scale approaches.

Interprofessional collaboration at the health and social care boundary

It is at the boundary between health and social care that some of the greatest challenges to interprofessional collaboration exist. This is also one of the most important areas for development. As the population of the UK, as in many other countries, becomes increasingly weighted towards older age, so the way in which society facilitates the effective care of older people becomes increasingly important. There are also still many challenges in creating an environment that supports people with disabilities and people with mental health problems in maximizing their quality of life. Policy changes in this area have already been described. With the advent of the NHS and Community Care Act, a formal partnership was established between health and social services. At the same time, many of the financial mechanisms previously relied upon were completely changed. Health authorities began to grapple with purchasing and commissioning health care for populations, defining more clearly what they were buying. Social services departments took on a new role as care managers, bringing together and managing the most appropriate package of care for each individual client. Somewhere between these two systems, one population based, the other mainly about individual need, many individual patients were lost (Jewell, 1993).

A new approach to the complexity of work at the boundaries between health and social care developed in Canada at McMaster University (Browne et al, 1996). It has been promoted in the UK by the King's Fund as the 'whole systems' approach. The theoretical underpinning of this is grounded in systems theory, which suggests that the whole is greater than the sum of its parts, and that 'rules' in complex systems may appear problematic only because most people look not at the whole system but only at their own part. A good example of the application of this approach in a complex system related to primary health care is the process of getting a patient home from hospital.

Patient discharge involves a very wide range of agencies and is frequently 'unsuccessful' for some of those involved. Unsuccessful discharges may range from those where the patient is kept in hospital for a lengthy period, long after they have recovered from the problem originally causing the admission, while a suitable placement is identified, to those where the patient is sent home at a few hours notice with inadequate information about his treatment and inadequate support for his carer. It was a discharge of the latter type that acted as the spur for a group in Newcastle upon Tyne to develop a whole systems event about going home from hospital (Newcastle Health Partnership, 1998).

Figure 4.1 shows the range of agencies identified in the event. The key components are health services (hospital and community based), including medical, nursing and paramedical services; local authority services, including social services and housing; and a variety of voluntary agencies. Some commercial organizations are also involved.

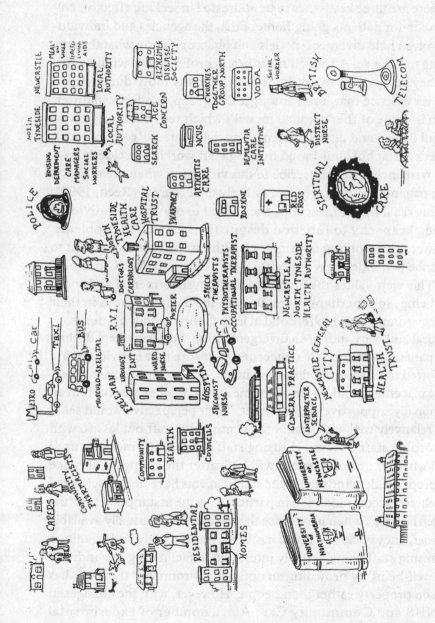

Figure 4.1: The range of agencies

For any individual patient or carer, tracking through the system may involve different players. Some, such as the GP, are frequently involved. Others, for example the speech therapist, may perhaps have much less association with the process of discharge.

There are three key issues to be addressed in seeking effective collaboration for patients going home. First, the agencies and individuals involved hold divergent models and philosophies on what they are seeking to achieve. Although most health professionals would agree that they are seeking to optimize health for any individual patient, there is evidence that, even amongst this group, models will differ. Much is made of the 'medical model', which sees health as a state without illness, and illness as something to be cured. Reed's research suggested that hospital-based nursing staff working in elderly care areas were inclined to subscribe to this view, even when the majority of the patients in their care were unlikely to be 'cured' (Reed, 1990). For this reason, she indicates, they failed to maximize individual patients' capacity to function despite their identified problems. However, staff working in primary health care appear more often to subscribe to a wider view of health, more allied to the WHO perspective. This view values the importance of physical, mental and social well-being, so is perhaps more likely to see the individuals in their own environment and to respond at least to their functional needs.

Local authority staff are a divergent group. Social workers dealing with patient discharge are concerned to ensure that individuals are supported to function optimally at home, or in an appropriate alternative placement, and, at least to some extent, that the patient is in an emotionally supportive environment. Their perspective would seem to fit relatively well with that of the community staff but less so with the hospital staff's views. Housing staff are perhaps more focused upon whether or not a tenant will look after the property or place inappropriate demands upon the staff. Patients have been discharged to sheltered accommodation in particular on the assumption that 'the warden is there', when in practice the warden is only usually available for emergency back-up. There has been, until recently, little tradition of housing staff being actively interested in facilitating any individual's well-being by providing an optimal environment: the focus has been on property rather than people. However, with the changes in the NHS and Community Care Act, a number of experimental schemes have been developed, by both local authorities and voluntary agencies, in which housing staff have worked with health and social care professionals to develop closer links and to support schemes to facilitate early discharge or indeed to avoid admission to hospital. Staff in voluntary agencies hold further, wide-ranging perspectives drawn from both health and social work contexts (Rodgers et al, 1997).

The second key issue to be addressed in seeking effective collaboration for patients going home is that the outcomes of the process desired, and indeed anticipated, by each of the players differ in nature. Some (usually professionals, and often quite senior ones) look primarily for quantitative outcomes: How many patients have been sent home? How long have they been in? How long has it taken to install this piece of equipment? How many visits have the patients had? The answers to these questions are factual. Other people (usually patients and carers but sometimes others) ask different questions: Why did she need to be in that long? Why did he not know when his mother would be discharged? Why could that couple not be enabled to achieve their goals? These questions uncover a more qualitative account of going home from hospital, one in which there are more contradictions. The speech therapist might, for example, feel that a stroke patient had been in too long, because he would have more opportunities to talk at home. The physiotherapist, on the other hand, might feel that a further period of concentrated work in hospital was desirable before discharge to a less intensive programme at home. Both professionals would be right, from their own perspectives, but different views could cause problems unless both were able to share their views.

Both types of outcome are important in planning and carrying out the discharge process. Without quantitative outcomes, it will not be possible to cost and organize the resources needed, yet without the qualitative outcomes, there will be only a relatively faint indication of the quality of the experience for any individual patient. In a complex process such as this, when professionals need to collaborate, it is important to enhance each group's recognition of the other's perspectives, so that each will collect appropriate data to support the others and each will negotiate a discharge plan that reflects all the patient's identified needs. Systems and structures must begin to be reconstructed to enable practitioners and managers to talk to each other about what they are trying to achieve.

Much of the discussion to date has reflected professional perspectives. However, consumer experience was central to the establishment of the whole system event in Newcastle. In relation to examining the quality of collaboration between agencies, as indicated earlier, consumers are in the strongest position to identify the holes in the safety net through which they fall. Thus the third issue is that we need to value and use consumer experience in developing agendas for collaboration and new and effective ways to collaborate. This is at the heart of the White Paper *The New NHS* (Secretary of State for Health, 1997b) and is discussed further in Chapter 9.

Ultimately, the process of going home from hospital is complex. The number of opportunities for collaboration is almost infinite. When different perspectives are taken into account and all outcomes are considered, successful discharge relies on three steps taking place in any collaboration. First, there must be adequate information transfer. Failures of communication are one of the most commonly cited reasons for poor or non-existent collaboration. Recent research (Pearson et al, 1998) indicates that records, which are often used as a medium of communication between different disciplines and different settings, are significantly inaccurate, with entries disagreeing between records for up to 26% of those analysed. Second, the participants must act appropriately on the information they have. To act appropriately, they need to understand the wider context in which they are acting and the roles of the other players. The same study indicates that professional participants often fail to act because they make inaccurate assumptions, for example about colleagues' roles or time scales for action, and that patients, too, influence the way in which professionals act. Third, some change must take place – the result or outcome of the action. For this to be recognized as a successful outcome, it should fit within the frameworks of one or more of the players.

Education for interprofessional collaboration

Although the importance of interprofessional training has been emphasized here and throughout this book, in practice it remains in its infancy. Research that has looked at education for interprofessional collaboration (Bryar, 1991; Horder, 1992; Vanclay, 1996) suggests that, in practice, little is done either before or after qualification to promote interprofessional collaboration, even between the core members of a primary health care team. Nevertheless, multiprofessional educational initiatives have been established throughout the UK, being more developed at continuing education level than undergraduate level.

Sigerist saw multiprofessional education as a means of removing doctors from their 'splendid isolation'. In 1943, Sigerist advised the Harvard Curriculum Committee that 'the students should be taught to work in teams' (Wislocki, 1943). This was an early step towards interprofessional training and the breaking down of insularity. Rather than focusing on making all health professionals experts in all areas, we should aim to establish a better understanding of what each profession has to offer and promote collaboration via interprofessional education:

> Today's disorders, falling to medical care ... are more frequently social health problems rather than disease specific, and not limited to the purview of a single profession for both diagnostic and therapeutic projections. (Miller and Rehr, 1983)

During the late 1980s and early 90s, a number of bodies were established with a particular interest in interprofessional education, including the Centre for the Advancement of Interprofessional Education in Primary Health and Community Care (CAIPE) and INTERACT. The Marylebone Centre Trust's Education and Training Unit was established in 1987, committed to a multidisciplinary approach to primary health care. Lessons learnt from Exeter University's pioneering interprofessional course have been reported elsewhere (Jones, 1986). In 1996, CAIPE surveyed the UK programmes (Barr and Waterton, 1996). Most of the courses they surveyed had been set up to meet common needs across professions (shared learning), but whilst professionals were increasingly learning together, there were limited opportunities to learn 'from and about one another'(interprofessional learning). Moreover, as highlighted by Leathard in her book *Going Inter-professional* (Leathard, 1994), interprofessional education lacks a theoretical basis.

As mentioned earlier, the 1996 policy documents explicitly recognized the multi-professionality of primary care. The White Paper *The National Health Service: A Service with Ambitions* (Secretary of State for Health, 1996b) specifically mentioned a long-term educational strategy. It highlighted the importance of shared learning, especially for continuing professional development, the accreditation of workplace learning, the need for widespread cultural change, the improvement of partnerships between patients and carers, the NHS, statutory and professional bodies and academic institutions and changes in funding, as well as the selection of appropriate students for a culture of lifelong learning, and the training and valuing of teachers with strong practice links.

With the shift from primary to secondary care in service provision, members of the primary health care team need to develop new skills and roles. In Chapter 5, Bond points to the under-utilization of the community pharmacist and foresees their increased involvement in

the primary health care team. As the membership of the primary
health care team extends, educational opportunities will need to be
reviewed. Educational processes need further consideration to promote appropriate, effective learning. A common credit system would
also facilitate shared learning initiatives.

An improved knowledge of one another's roles and a better understanding of the underpinning concepts and philosophies are vital.
Divergent models can explain the different goal expectations across
groups. For example, Ross (Chapter 3) discusses concerns that nurses
might lose their more holistic 'caring' approach should they adopt the
traditional medical 'cure' model. How can such a diversity of views be
addressed to enable effective collaboration? In the main, it seems most
appropriately addressed through education. Knowledge, attitudes and
behaviour are to be influenced. At undergraduate or pre-registration
level, students must be made aware of the range of perspectives and
priorities that exist, and should be taught to value each other's views.
Once qualified, practitioners from all disciplines need opportunities
from time to time to reflect further on the beliefs and values of their colleagues, the ways in which these may impact on their handling of various situations in practice and the ways in which this may affect their
own practice. Multiprofessional education and training should aim to
promote the best components of the respective professions and minimize threats to professional insecurity and competency. Equal status
has to be promoted for interprofessional collaboration to succeed
(Dingwall and McIntosh, 1978).

Some of the various theories that inform collaboration were highlighted above. An appreciation of such academic principles should be
a pre-requisite to effective collaborative working. Principles of teamworking and skills could be taught on an interprofessional basis at
undergraduate/pre-registration level. Continuing interprofessional
education may take the form of joint training for GPs and practice
nurses, or primary and secondary care-based workers developing
specialist roles, for example in palliative care and mental health.
There is scope for educational partnerships between GPs, community/
practice pharmacists and nurses via joint protocols for prescribing.
Being a care provider involves organizational skills; integrated nurse
and other teams can be actively educated via guidelines and protocols
to adopt a systems-based approach to work.

Nor is it simply a matter of educating professionals together.
We must see education in the context of the increased workload in
primary care. We cannot burden people further by imposing imprac-
tical educational structures upon them. We have already observed the

negative impact of the market approach upon morale. New means of structuring education are therefore required. There is a need for further innovations such as the Liverpool and Team Valleys projects, where shared learning occurred in its broadest sense, with practitioners learning via development and evaluation projects while remaining firmly in their clinical areas.

Conclusion

This chapter has examined some of the policy shifts that are increasingly encouraging interprofessional collaboration, with particular reference to the NHS and Community Care Act, the Primary Care Act and its associated White Papers and planned changes in NHS structure. Some of the ways in which collaboration occurs in primary health care practice were outlined. Models and theories of interprofessional collaboration have been discussed and linked to research in a range of primary health care settings. Interprofessional collaboration was explored in a complex system – the discharge of patients from hospital. The importance of interprofessional education was considered. Three key issues were identified in promoting collaboration: first, the need to build on, and where possible combine, divergent models and philosophies; second, the need to draw together and value both quantitative and qualitative outcomes; and finally, the need to incorporate consumer perspectives in developing agendas for collaboration and effective ways of collaborating.

References

Armitage P (1983) Joint working in primary health care. Nursing Times 79: 75–8.

Barr H, Waterton S (1996) Summary of a CAIPE survey: interprofessional education in health and social care in the United Kingdom. Journal of Interprofessional Care 10: 297–303.

Belbin R M (1981) Management Teams: Why They Succeed or Fail. London: Heinemann.

Belbin R M (1993) Team Roles at Work. London: Butterworth–Heinemann.

Bennett-Emslie G, McIntosh J (1995) Promoting collaboration in the primary care team – the role of the practice meeting. Journal of Interprofessional Care 9: 251–6.

Black S, Hagel D (1995) Working together in primary care: an integrated team approach. Health Visitor 69: 280–3.

Brown I (1997) A skill mix parent support initiative in health visiting: an evaluation study. Health Visitor 70: 339–43.

Browne G, Watt S, Roberts J, Gafni A, Byrne C (1996) Within our Reach: Restructuring Alliances in Health and Social Services at the Local Level. Hamilton, Ontario: McMaster University.

Bryar R (1991) Primary Health Care Teamwork Education in Wales: An Exploratory Study. Cardiff: Teamcare Valleys.

Bryar R, Bytheway B (1996) Changing Primary Health Care. The Teamcare Valleys Experience. Oxford: Blackwell.

Carlisley D (1993) From hospital to community. Nursing Times 89: 37–9.

Concise Oxford Dictionary, 5th Edn (1990) Oxford: Oxford University Press.

Department of Health (1998) Our Healthier Nation. London: HMSO.

Department of Health and Social Security (1974) Annual Report. London: HMSO.

Department of Health and the Welsh Office (1989) General Practice in the National Health Service: A New Contract. London: HMSO.

Dingwall R, McIntosh J (1978) Teamwork in theory and practice. In Dingwall R, McIntosh J, Readings in the Sociology of Nursing. Edinburgh: Churchill Livingstone.

Dyer W (1987) Teambuilding: Issues and Alternatives. Chicago: Addison-Wesley.

Edward S (1997) Working in the wider team. In Pearson P, Spencer J (Eds) Promoting Teamwork in Primary Care: A Research Based Approach. London: Arnold.

Finlay F (1998) Providing healthcare information suitable for adolescents. Health Visitor 71: 16–18.

Gilley M (1996) Collaboration between Health and Social Services for the Implementation of Community Care. Sunderland: University of Sunderland.

Glasman D (1993) Things that go bump in the night. Health Service Journal 103: 16.

Gregson B, Cartlidge A, Bond J (1991) Interprofessional Collaboration in Primary Health Care Organisations. Occasional Paper 52, London: RCGP.

Horder J (1992) CAIPE: a national survey that needs to be repeated. Journal of Interprofessional Care 6: 65–71.

Hudson H, Bennett G (1997) Action research: a vehicle for change in general practice? In Pearson P, Spencer J (Eds) Promoting Teamwork in Primary Care: A Research Based Approach. London: Arnold.

Jewell S (1993) Discovery of the discharge process: a study of patient discharge from a care unit for elderly people. Journal of Advanced Nursing 18: 1288–96.

Jones R V H (1986) Working Together, Learning Together. Occasional Paper No. 33. London: RCGP.

Jowell T (1997) Keynote speech, Health Strategy Conference. Target 25: 5–7.

Leathard A (1994) Going Inter-professional: Working Together for Health and Welfare. London: Routledge.

Meethan K F (1995) Empowerment and community care for older people. In Nelson N, Wright S (Eds) Power and Participatory Development. London: Intermediate Technology Publications.

Miller R S, Rehr H (1983) Health settings and health providers. In Miller R

S, Rehr H (Eds) Social Work Issues in Health Care. New Jersey: Prentice-Hall.

National Health Service Executive (1997) Health Action Zones – Invitation to Bid. EL(97)65. London: HMSO.

Nazareth I, King M, SeeTai S (1997) Monitoring psychosis in general practice: a controlled trial. British Journal of Psychiatry 169: 475–82.

Newcastle Health Partnership (1998) The Going Home Common Strategy. Newcastle: Newcastle City Council.

Niven N (1994) Health Psychology, 2nd Edn. Edinburgh: Churchill Livingstone.

O'Gorman F (1996) Community development: innovation in practice. In Twinn S, Roberts B, Andrews S (Eds) Community Health Care Nursing: Principles for Practice. Oxford: Butterworth–Heinemann.

Øvretveit J (1995) Coordinating Community Care. Buckingham: Open University Press.

Pearson P (1997) Evaluating teambuilding In Pearson P, Spencer J (Eds) Promoting Teamwork in Primary Care: A Research Based Approach. London: Arnold.

Pearson P, Procter S, Wilcockson J, Haighton K, Spendiff A, Allgar V (1998) Discharging Patients Effectively: Planning for Best Care. Newcastle upon Tyne: University of Newcastle.

Pearson P, van Zwanenberg T (1991) Who Is the Primary Health Care Team? What Should They be Doing? Newcastle upon Tyne: University of Newcastle.

Poulton B, West M (1994) Primary health care team effectiveness: developing a constituency approach. Health and Social Care in the Community 2: 77–84.

Reed J (1990) All dressed up and nowhere to go. Newcastle: CNAA, Newcastle Polytechnic.

Ringelmann M (1913) Recherches sur les moreurs animes: travail de l'homme. Annales de l'Institut National Agronomique 1–40.

Rodgers H, Souther J, Kaiser W et al (1997) Early supported hospital discharge following acute stroke: length of stay and three month outcomes. Clinical Rehabilitation 11: 280–7.

Royal College of Nursing (1980) Primary Health Care Nursing – A Team Approach. London: RCN.

Secretary of State for Health (1992) The Health of the Nation: A Strategy for Health in England. London: HMSO.

Secretary of State for Health (1996a) Primary Care: The Future – Choice and Opportunity. London: HMSO.

Secretary of State for Health (1996b) The National Health Service: A Service with Ambitions. London: HMSO.

Secretary of State for Health (1996c) Primary Care: Delivering the Future. London: HMSO.

Secretary of State for Health (1997a) The New NHS. London: HMSO.

Secretary of State for Health (1997b) Developing Partnerships in Mental Health. London: HMSO.

Smith A, Melville E (1996) Targeting teenagers in the primary health care setting. Health Visitor 69(6): 228–30.

Spratley J (1989) Disease Prevention and Health Promotion in Primary

Care: An Evaluation Report. Oxford: Health Education Authority.

Stacy R, Christian F, Drinkwater C (1996) Evaluation of a Pilot Study to Place a Welfare Rights Service in General Practice. Newcastle upon Tyne: University of Newcastle.

Standing Medical Advisory Committee and Standing Nursing and Midwifery Advisory Committee (1981) The Primary Health Care Team: Report of a Joint Working Group (Harding Committee). London: HMSO.

Stilwell B, Greenfield S, Drury V, Hull F (1987) A nurse practitioner in general practice: working styles and pattern of consultations. Journal of the Royal College of General Practitioners 37: 154–7.

Thomas P, Graver L (1997) The Liverpool intervention to promote teamwork in general practice: an action research approach. In Pearson P, Spencer J (Eds) Promoting Teamwork in Primary Care: A Research Based Approach. London: Arnold.

Usherwood T, Long S, Joesbury H (1997) The changing composition of primary health care teams. In Pearson P, Spencer J (Eds) Promoting Teamwork in Primary Care: A Research Based Approach. London: Arnold.

Vanclay L (1996) Sustaining collaboration between general practitioners and social workers. London: Centre for the Advancement of Interprofessional Education.

Weich S, Lewis G, Churchill R, Mann A (1997) Strategies for the prevention of psychiatric disorder in primary care in South London. Journal of Epidemiology and Community Health 51: 304–9.

Weldon E, Weingart L R (1993) Group goals and group performance. British Journal of Social Psychology 32: 307–34.

West M, Poulton B (1997a) Defining and measuring effectiveness for primary health care teams In Pearson P, Spencer J (Eds) Promoting Teamwork in Primary Care: A Research Based Approach. London: Arnold.

West M, Poulton B (1997b) Primary health care teams: in a league of their own. In Pearson P, Spencer J (Eds) Promoting Teamwork in Primary Care: A Research Based Approach. London: Arnold.

Wislocki G B (1943) Meeting of the Curriculum Committee on the Presentation to it by Sigerist Oct 27 1943. Papers of the Harvard School of Medicine, the Francis A Countway Library of Medicine.

Woodhouse K, Macmahon D, Williams R (1997) Services for People who are Elderly. Norwich: HMSO.

World Health Organisation (1978) Primary Health Care: Report of the International Conference on Primary Health Care, Alma-Ata, USSR 1978. Geneva: WHO.

Young G (1996) Counsellors are seeing people with previously unmet needs. British Medical Journal 313: 1208.

Zito J (1994) Watching brief. Nursing Times 90: 18.

Chapter 5
Pharmacy and primary health care

Christine Bond

Introduction

There are currently over 30 000 registered pharmacists practising in Great Britain, and the majority – 21 000 – work in community pharmacies that are either single outlets, small chains or one of a small number of major multiples. Proprietors of these premises are independent contractors to the NHS. Since the establishment of the NHS, the main contribution of pharmacy to primary health care has been through the dispensing of prescriptions (written by doctors, dentists, veterinary practitioners and more recently selected nurses) and the provision of advice on minor ailments, accompanied by the sale of appropriate medication. In order to ensure a comprehensive network of community pharmacies at a minimal cost, it was always intended that NHS remuneration, which is largely related to the dispensing role, would be supplemented by such commercial activity.

Pharmacists are regulated by their own professional body, the Royal Pharmaceutical Society of Great Britain (RPSGB), and governed by its Code of Ethics. Entry to the profession is through successful completion of a 4-year university course, leading to the degree of Master of Pharmacy, and a year of pre-registration training followed by a final entry examination. A large number of pharmacists hold additional specialized higher degrees in clinical pharmacy.

There is a recognition that pharmacy is an undervalued profession and that pharmacists are over-trained for what they actually do and under-utilized given what they know (Eaton and Webb, 1979). This is particularly so in comparison with the status of the profession in some other countries, for example France, where pharmacy has developed as one of the great professions (Trease, 1965). There is clear evidence that the status of the profession in the hospital context has increased since the parallel increase in its clinical role (Smith and Knapp, 1972; Cotter et al, 1994). There is now a general awareness at national level that there should be an equivalent increased utilization of the pharmacist in primary care, although clear differences, such as ease of access to the prescriber (Barber et al, 1994), may result in the development of different models of pharmaceutical care. The need for this to include greater interaction with the patient is illustrated by the following quotation:

> Those in leadership positions in academic pharmacy recognize that their profession's upward mobility in the academic pecking order is related to more direct involvement of pharmacists in patient care. (Morris, 1980)

In this chapter, selected key issues are surveyed from the perspectives of the pharmaceutical and medical professions, with consideration of the implications for the patient and the NHS.

Background

Historical background

GPs and pharmacists have a common ancestor in the mediaeval spicers, who formed themselves into the Society of Apothecaries in 1617. They were in competition with the physicians, who by royal decree were the only group licensed to give, and charge for, medical advice (Eaton and Webb, 1979). It was the apothecaries' task both to dispense medicines for physicians and to recommend medicines for those members of the public unable to afford physicians' fees. However, they were not themselves permitted to charge for this advice. In 1815, the Apothecaries Act allowed a charge to be made specifically for the giving of advice as well as for the medicine that was dispensed (Matthews, 1980), and, as a result of subsequent legislation, the two distinct professions of pharmacy and general practice medicine emerged, the main role of the community pharmacist increasingly becoming that of dispenser.

The main argument for maintaining the two professions of medicine and pharmacy, and thereby separating the prescribing and dispensing functions, has been the acknowledged conflict that would otherwise exist when income is related to the quantity and cost of the medicine prescribed. For example, in Japan, where the doctor is commonly responsible for both prescribing and dispensing (Macarthur, 1992; Takemasa, 1994), drug costs are higher than anywhere else in the world, and 30% of the total expenditure on health is spent on drugs (Axon, 1994), amounting to $228 per person per year compared with $169 Germany, the second highest spender (*Economist*, 1993). However, unlike the rest of Europe, where the two professions are historically distinct, dispensing doctors are virtually unknown and pharmacists enjoy a high professional standing that is the envy of their British colleagues (Trease, 1965), UK pharmacists never quite achieved a monopoly over dispensing (Matthews, 1980), and dispensing doctors are still fairly common. Published figures for England and Wales indicate that the costs of drugs dispensed by dispensing doctors is higher than that for doctors who only prescribe (Bond, 1994a; Prescription Pricing Authority, 1994).

Official papers and recommendations

Encouragement has been given to those believing that community pharmacists could play a greater part in the delivery of primary health care by a series of government publications (Table 5.1), some focusing on pharmacy, others considering the overall delivery of health care.

Recognition that the profession of pharmacy was no longer being utilized to its full potential, because of external factors, was first officially identified in 1979 (Merrison, 1979). Following this, the Nuffield report in 1986 clearly identified that community pharmacists could play a more central role in health care delivery (Nuffield Foundation, 1986). The Nuffield report was particularly important

Table 5.1: Key reports including recommendations for community pharmacy

Date	Report	Remit
1979	Report on the NHS (HMSO) Royal Commission on the National Health Service	The best use and management of the financial and manpower resources of the NHS
1986	Pharmacy: Report to the Nuffield Foundation	Consideration of the present and future structure of pharmacy, its contribution to health care, its education and training
1987	Promoting Better Health (HMSO)	Proposals to improve primary health care and the services offered to patients

(contd)

Table 5.1: (contd)

Date	Report	Remit
1989	Role and Function of the Pharmacist in Europe (WHO)	A definition of the functions and responsibilities of the pharmacist in the health care system of an industrialized country and recommendations for further development
1989	Working for Patients (HMSO)	Proposals to give patients better health care and a greater choice of services, to give greater satisfaction and rewards for those working in the NHS who respond to local needs
1992	Pharmaceutical Care: The Future for Community Pharmacy (DoH)	Consideration of ways in which the NHS community pharmaceutical services might be developed to increase their contribution to health care and to make recommendations
1992	Community Pharmacies in England (NAO)	The economy, efficiency and effectiveness of community pharmacy
1996	Primary Care: Choice and Opportunity (HMSO)	An exploration of novel working relationships in primary care with a special chapter for pharmacy
1997	Agenda for Action (HMSO)	A detailed summary of possible regulatory and logistical mechanisms for implementing a primary care-led NHS
1996	The New Horizon (Royal Pharmaceutical Society of Great Britain)	Report of a widespread consultation within the profession to review the status of the profession and make decisions for the future
1997	Building the Future (Royal Pharmaceutical Society of Great Britain)	Summary of examples and proposals to implement the wider role for community pharmacy

because it was seen to be an objective pronouncement by opinion-formers outside the profession who would have little, if any, vested interest in its recommendations.

The overall message of the Nuffield Foundation was embraced in the context of general health care with the publication of the White Paper *Promoting Better Health* (Department of Health, 1987). This was not specifically about a policy for pharmacy but about an overall NHS policy for the future, aimed at the optimization of existing resources, in the broadest sense, at a time when public expectations of health care were continuing to rise but could not easily be met out of current resource allocations.

A further significant publication was the joint policy document of the Department of Health and the RPSGB (1992), *Pharmaceutical Care: The Future for Community Pharmacy*, which concentrated specifically on the future role of the community pharmacist and was based on extensive consultation both within and outside the profession. This document considered various aspects of the community pharmacist's working practice under nine broad headings, including services to GPs, the over-the-counter (OTC) advisory role, health promotion, and services to special needs groups such as the housebound. Thirty specific tasks listed in the document's annexe were recommended to be introduced either nationally or on a pilot basis. Whilst some of these tasks merely formalized ongoing practice and were generally welcomed, others were very innovative, covering diverse areas from simple health care advice to therapeutic drug monitoring, and prescribing following agreed protocols. ('Prescribing' has been defined, in the Collins *Concise English Dictionary*, as a recommendation for the use of a drug or remedy.) The report was received with some reservations by medical bodies (*Pharmaceutical Journal*, 1992a) but was welcomed as 'pragmatic, prosaic, and progressive' by the pharmaceutical profession (*Pharmaceutical Journal*, 1992b, 1992c).

Most recently, two further key publications affecting the contribution of pharmacy to primary health care have been published. *Primary Care: The Future – Choice and Opportunity* (Secretary of State for Health, 1996), one of the first White Papers to address primary care, had a separate chapter dedicated to pharmacy. It was followed by *Primary Care: Agenda for Action* (Scottish Office Department of Health, 1997), which identified mechanisms and remuneration for implementing changes that would integrate the pharmacist into the core, as opposed to the peripheral, primary health care team. Also in 1996, the profession undertook a wide consultation amongst its members to agree a future role for the profession, an initiative known as the New Age. It culminated in the publication of a key document, *The New Horizon: A Consultation on the Future of the Profession*, which detailed four key areas for pharmacists to contribute to care and was followed a year later by *Building the Future*, which used examples of innovative practice to propose ways of translating strategy into practice (Royal Pharmaceutical Society of Great Britain, 1996, 1997a).

The community pharmacist and the primary health care team

It has long been this author's belief that the community pharmacist is under-utilized and is not recognized as a peer by other health care professionals, yet has the potential to contribute more to primary health care and to the primary health care team. The primary health care team was first described in 1979 by the Royal Commission on the NHS (Merrison, 1979). Almost a decade later, Drury (1988) commented, 'one thing that can be said about team work in general practice is that there is not a lot of it about'. The implicit requirement for GPs to delegate to other members of the primary health care team was thus slow to be implemented. However, there is evidence that this has changed dramatically in recent years, probably motivated by radical changes in the delivery of NHS care. Yet, unlike other paramedical groups and professions, the community pharmacist is still not seen to be part of the primary health care team, certainly not part of the core team and often not part of the wider team (Martin, 1992). This does not reflect the wishes of the profession. A survey of community pharmacists in two FHSAs in England showed that 95% were overwhelmingly in favour of being part of a multi-disciplinary primary health care team (Sutters and Nathan, 1993).

A survey of London community pharmacists carried out in the late 1980s showed frequent contact with the GP, but the vast majority of contacts were associated with prescriptions, and three-quarters of these contacts were initiated by the pharmacist (Smith, 1990). Forty-three per cent had some contact with primary health care personnel other than GPs; of these, the most frequently cited professionals were the district nurse and the staff of residential homes, although 17 different professionals were named, and the contacts were mostly initiated by the other profession rather than the pharmacist. The frequency of contact was at least weekly, yet 60% of the responding pharmacists felt that, in spite of this level of contact, their contribution to the team was not acknowledged.

There are many ways in which the community pharmacist could play a greater part in the primary health care team, with respect to both prescribed and non-prescribed medication, at interfaces with the GP and other health care professionals, and with the public (Department of Health and Royal Pharmaceutical Society of Great Britain, 1992; Cox, 1993). The needs of the patient will be central to these interactions, which may cause problems for the pharmacist when the patient's needs appear to conflict with the GP's instructions. This anomalous, two-faceted role – carrying out the prescribing instructions of GPs, yet with direct access to the patient population, who may consult the pharmacist directly – is in contrast to the historical position of other health care professionals such as nurses.

GPs have been found to support a wider role for the community pharmacist, as suggested by the recent reports, although certain more radical proposals, for example therapeutic drug monitoring, have, to date, received little support (Bond et al, 1995). Roles that were supported tended to be skewed towards technical drug distribution and information provision and away from clinical interaction with the patient with respect to prescribed medication. The wider 'over-the-counter' role, enhanced by an increased armamentarium of drugs that the community pharmacist can recommend or prescribe, was supported by just under half of the GPs, yet this is now established practice (see below). The reasons for negative attitudes appeared to be associated with traditional professional boundaries, hierarchies and paternalistic feelings amongst GPs towards 'their' patients.

The current extended primary care role

Published evidence reports that some pharmacists are adopting innovative practices with the support of their local GP, for example therapeutic drug monitoring (Harrison, 1992; Hawksworth, 1992; Wells, 1992; Maguire and McElnay, 1993) and formulary advice (Roddick et al, 1993); there are other examples supported by health authorities, for example health education (Todd, 1993). There have been many recent reports of pharmacists working in general practice surgeries to interpret computerized prescribing reports (PACT in England and SPA in Scotland), to review computerized repeat prescription records and to run special disease clinics to consider areas such as dyspepsia and its appropriate treatment, or anticoagulation clinics. Demand for such primary care pharmacists is increasing in parallel with an awareness of their valuable input (Weir et al, 1997), although there is often a mismatch between what pharmacists would like to do and what GPs would like them to do (Jesson et al, 1997)! There has been a proliferation of courses specifically addressing the needs of this group of pharmacists, who come from both hospital and community backgrounds, both updating on therapeutics and informing on other general practice issues such as prescription data feedback (PACT/SPA) and general practice computer systems.

Benefits of the extended role

Six million people are reputed to visit a pharmacy every day (Department of Health and Royal Pharmaceutical Society, 1992). The pharmacy is seen as a 'high street health shop' (Lewis, 1994), and the pharmacist is always accessible without an appointment (Smith, 1992). Thus the potential benefits for primary care of a wider pharmaceutical role to the public are clear.

Most people visit a pharmacy to purchase either prescribed or non-prescribed medicine, and public consumption of drugs is steadily increasing irrespective of social class. In a major study of the general population, 80% of adults and 55% of children had taken at least one medicine in the preceding 2 weeks, two-thirds of which were non-prescribed (Dunnell, 1973). More recent figures confirm that sales of OTC medicines have increased at the rate of almost 2% annually over the past 5 years, the two largest areas being cough and cold remedies, followed closely by analgesics (Datamonitor, 1992; Proprietary Association of Great Britain, 1994). A valuable contribution from the community pharmacist is in ensuring that these medicines are taken appropriately, through their safety net role when dispensing against a prescription, informed by the computerized patient records that they keep for the majority of patients and by the supervision of sales of the more potent OTC medicines. Thus drug interactions can be identified and the prescriber/customer alerted, and adverse drug reactions can be reported and contraindications avoided.

The recent Audit Office report on community pharmacies (National Audit Office, 1992) says that community pharmacists are already fulfilling vital roles in relation to the NHS yet only account for 2% of its overall budget. The auditors believe that the contribution of community pharmacy to health care may evolve to become even more central in the next decade. Tasks that they highlight include generic substitution, extended patient medication records, further 'depomming' (the deregulation of medicines from prescription-only medicine – POM – to pharmacy-supervised medicine – P; see below), involvement in screening and health education, discretion in repeat prescribing, domiciliary services, therapeutic drug monitoring and improved professional advice.

Thus, from the 'high street' premises, the pharmacist could be seen as helping the GP indirectly by providing advice from community pharmacies for patients who would otherwise consult the doctor for trivial or minor ailments. Whilst it must be remembered that such a definition is *post hoc* and possibly only confirmed after medical differentiation, such consultations have been estimated to constitute a third or even a half of all patients seen by GPs (Cartwright and Anderson, 1981).

Within the general practice setting, the benefits of a pharmacy input are in advice to GPs on formulary development, the interpretation of PACT/SPA feedback, the rationalization of therapy, the monitoring of repeat prescribing and involvement in disease clinics. These developments are still relatively new and as yet largely unevaluated other than as case studies of a single centre.

Legislative changes

Many of the changes proposed for pharmacy will require regulatory and legislative changes to implement them. An example of one such change that has already been introduced is the deregulation of medicines.

Deregulation of medicines

The constantly increasing expenditure on health care has posed a currently unresolved problem for Western nations over the past few decades, and governments have looked at various ways of reducing these costs. A reduction in the primary care drugs bill is one such target, and community pharmacists are expected to become more involved in the future in two areas: repeat prescribing and OTC advice, that is, pharmaceutical support for self-care.

Self-care is a cost-effective component of all health care systems whether they are private or national (see Chapter 9 for a further discussion of self-care). The full potential has been limited to date because of legal restrictions on the range of drugs that are available for sale, restricting many to POM status. Recent government-led moves have increased the number of such drugs by a deregulation process that has been termed 'depomming' by the Medicines Control Agency (see above). This parallels worldwide moves to increase the availability of a wider range of medicines so that 'no medicine should remain POM unless necessary for reasons of safety'. This became a European Community directive for medicines classification (92/26/CEE) and the basis on which further medicines have been deregulated.

The process started slowly in the UK with the deregulation of ibuprofen and loperamide (1983), terfenadine (1984) and hydrocortisone 1% cream (1985) but has continued steadily with the support of the government (Bottomley, 1989), the RPSGB (Department of Health and Royal Pharmaceutical Society of Great Britain, 1992; Royal Pharmaceutical Society of Great Britain, 1995), individual pharmacists (Bond et al, 1993) and, to a limited extent, the Royal College of General Practitioners (Royal College of General Practitioners, 1993). A list of the recently deregulated or depommed medicines in the UK is shown in Table 5.2. Other target preparations for future deregulation include oral contraceptives and the 'morning after' pill (Drife, 1993; *Lancet*, 1993), which has the support of both the Royal College of General Practitioners (1995) and the General Medical Services Committee of the British Medical Association (1995).

Economic considerations

An OTC purchase of drugs can save patients money as well as their time and opportunity costs. Patients are saved the costs of visiting the doctor followed by a visit to the pharmacist. For those patients who would normally pay a prescription charge, the savings will depend on the price of the deregulated product, but if the patient is normally exempt from the prescription charge, the only savings are the indirect non-drug costs. Where costs are defined to include both monetary and non-monetary elements, figures show that the OTC availability of topical 1% hydrocortisone saved patients £2 million in 1987 alone (Ryan and Yule, 1988, 1990). The use of standard economic models of supply and demand can also be shown to demonstrate the theoretical economic advantages to the NHS of switching to OTC medications (Ryan and Bond, 1994).

A prospective study of advice contacts where the community pharmacist would like to recommend a currently POM product indicated that most of the presenting symptoms could already be treated by currently available P medicines (Bond et al, 1995). This suggests that the effect of deregulation could be purely to make available more effective treatments for symptoms about which the public consult the pharmacist anyway, rather than to increase the number of such con-

Table 5.2: A chronological list of medicines whose UK status has changed from prescription only to pharmacy supervised

Date	Ingredient	Date	Ingredient
1983	ibuprofen	1993	tioconazole (vaginal)
	loperamide		nicotine 4 mg gum
1984	terfenadine		hydrocortisone (oral pellet)
1985	hydrocortisone 1% (topical)		aluminium chloride
			hexahydrate (topical)
1986	miconazole	1994	diclofenac (topical)
1988	ibuprofen sr and topical		felbinac (topical)
1989	astemizole		piroxicam (topical)
	mebendazole		flunisolide (nasal spray)
	dextromethorphan		ranitidine
1991	nicotine 2 mg gum		minoxidil (topical)
1992	hyoscine N-butyl bromide		Adcortyl in Orabase
	nicotine patches		Anusol Plus HC ointment
	vaginal imidazoles		Anusol Plus HC
	hydrocortisone with		suppositories
	crotamiton (topical)	1995	hydroxyzine hydrochloride
	carbenoxolone		pyrantel embonate
	paracetamol and		fluconazole
	dihydrocodeine		ketoconazole (topical)
1993	loratidine		hydrocortisone rectal
	aciclovir (topical)		cadexomer iodine
	acrivastine		budesonide nasal
	cetirizine	1996	azelastine nasal
	ketoprofen (topical)		nizatidine
	cimetidine		hydrocortisone/lignocaine
	famotidine		perianal spray
	beclomethasone dipropionate		mebeverine hydrochloride
	(nasal)		aciclovir, additional named
	mebendazole (multiple dose)		products
	pseudoephedrine sr		clotrimazole with
	sodium cromoglycate		hydrocortisone
	(ophthalmic)		

Data from Royal Pharmaceutical Society of Great Britain (1997b).

tacts. However, if recently deregulated products such as clotrimazole and beclomethasone nasal spray are considered, once a product is available over the counter, and the public is made aware of this by the accompanying advertising, the demand for an OTC purchase of that product will increase, as happened with the anti-ulcer drugs discussed below.

Drugs used for the treatment of minor, acute self-limiting disease may be expected largely to disappear from prescribing statistics. An example of this sort of drug would be topical aciclovir (Zovirax), used in the treatment of herpes labialis (cold sores). However, a possibly more complex picture could evolve with drugs such as the H_2 blockers, which are generally marketed at a lower dose than their POM counterparts (raising concerns about efficacy) and which can be used to treat long-term symptoms that may or may not indicate serious diseases.

The purchase of H_2 blockers to treat transient dyspepsia will result in a shift of the drug distribution mechanism from general practice to the community pharmacist and the public. The longer-term implication could be a greater volume of prescribed H_2 blockers as the public learn of the existence of an effective treatment yet are not prepared to pay in the long term for it. (Also, the community pharmacist should not allow long-term use if supervising sales in accordance with the P licence.) Second, the fact that less effective doses are being purchased may mean that the GP, faced with a patient who has received no benefit from an H_2 blocker (the first-line treatment), may go straight to the second-line, more expensive prescription (the proton pump inhibitor). This is not because the GP is unaware of the difference but because, on balance, he chooses to prescribe the treatment more likely to be effective rather than chance an intermediate approach, which, should it be ineffective, would result in the need for a second consultation.

Feasibility studies and future research

Feasibility studies

Many of the roles discussed above have been the subject of research. Whilst much of this research has been criticized for being restricted to small pilot studies (Mays, 1994) that do not meet the grade 1 evidence required by, for example, the Cochrane Collaboration (a randomized controlled trial conducted according to the strictest criteria), it is useful in demonstrating the feasibility of the proposals.

Health promotion

Much work has been conducted to demonstrate the potential contribution of the community pharmacist to smoking cessation. In the most rigorous study yet, using a randomized controlled design, Sinclair et al (1998) demonstrated that pharmacists and their assistants who had undergone 2 hours of specific training in behavioural change could significantly increase the smoking cessation rate of their customers, from 7% to 12%. This success rate is comparable to that of many other medical interventions and was shown to be extremely cost-effective.

Repeat prescribing

Current problems in repeat prescribing have been highlighted by the National Audit Office (1993) and others (Harris and Dajda, 1996; Zermansky, 1996). Repeat prescribing accounts for over 70% of all dispensed items and has been associated with inadequate clinical review, the stockpiling of unwanted medicines, inappropriate polypharmacy and poor compliance. All of these have direct and indirect cost implications for the NHS.

The community pharmacist can help to address all of the above problems if given the discretion to review patients' needs against an agreed protocol on a monthly basis. This has been demonstrated to be acceptable to patients and GPs, to result in an average cost avoidance of £22 per patient and to identify compliance or drug-related problems in 12% of patients (Bond et al, 1998a).

In the general practice setting and prior to dispensing, pharmacists can review patient records, identify high-risk patients on polypharmacy regimes and check on drug interactions, contraindications and concordance. Compliance with local formulary policy can also be checked (Krska, personal communication, 1997).

Disease management

In one general practice, a pharmacist used computerized records to identify all patients on long-term anti-ulcer drugs. In a clinic-based setting, patients were invited to attend, and their need for long-term therapy was reviewed. Many were found not to have an indication for anti-ulcer treatment, and many with diagnosed ulcers had not received the recommended eradication therapy. As a result, 90% of the practice's dyspepsia patients benefited, and savings of £380 000 were achieved (Royal Pharmaceutical Society of Great Britain, 1997a). New patients presenting with dyspepsia have also been treated in a way which has resulted in cost avoidance compared with standard practice (MacIntyre et al, 1997).

Dyspepsia-type symptoms can also be treated appropriately through OTC purchases that can be integrated with practice-based action to provide a co-ordinated approach to treatment. Clinical guidelines have recently been developed for dyspepsia by a multidisciplinary group. Pharmacists' knowledge increased through use of these guidelines, and patients accepted the structured questioning imposed by the guidelines (Bond et al, 1998b).

Domiciliary visits

Domiciliary visits by pharmacists to selected patients, by agreement with the GP, have also been demonstrated to be of value (Williams et al, 1996). In a small sample of 117 patients, pharmacists identified problems related to drug interactions between prescribed and non-prescribed medication, drug side-effects, formulation, packaging and labelling problems. This type of service is particularly important for elderly patients, who are often unable to visit the pharmacy themselves and therefore do not benefit from direct pharmaceutical input when collecting their medicines.

Services to drug misusers

The treatment of drug misusers is an escalating problem, and drug misuse is associated with huge social consequences of crime and the spread of blood-borne diseases. Current strategies are based on a harm minimization approach, which for pharmacy involves selling or exchanging needles and syringes, and supervising the consumption of prescribed substitute methadone. Interviews with drug misusers show the importance of pharmacists in contributing to the success of the programmes through providing consistent advice and preventing leakage on to the illicit market. In Glasgow, where pharmacists and GPs have collaborated and almost all methadone consumption is now supervised on pharmacy premises following agreed guidelines, the success of the programme is demonstrated by a documented reduction in drug-related crime and a reduction in the number of needle exchanges (Matheson, 1998).

Future research

An awareness of the limitations of much of the recent research into the practice of pharmacy led the RPSGB, together with the King's Fund to convene a Pharmacy Practice Research and Development Task Force. Their report, *Investing in Evidence-based Practice in Pharmacy* (Royal Pharmaceutical Society of Great Britain and King's

Fund, 1997) highlights the new opportunities for pharmacists in primary care and the need to demonstrate through research that any new service is cost-effective and based on sound evidence. Pharmacy is said to be 'one of the most complex but least analysed of the health care services'. Research 'has to have a clear focus and address the right issues in the right way, be of high quality, have a solid funding base, and a culture of research awareness must be fostered amongst all practising pharmacists' (Royal Pharmaceutical Society of Great Britain and King's Fund, 1996). The report recommended that pharmacy practice research be predominantly multi-disciplinary, use a range of methods and be carried out jointly by academics and practitioners, in the context of the wider multiprofessional delivery of health care. The report endorses that the whole profession should be users of research, with a proportion doing research and a small minority leading research.

To address the right questions to support the extended primary care role, the Task Force recommends that research considers the following essential subject areas:

- the structure, organization, functions and responsibilities, and process of pharmacy;
- the beliefs, expectations, needs and outcomes of patients and other professionals;
- the development, supply and distribution, usage and management of medicines.

Barriers and incentives to change

Whilst the opportunities to implement a wider role are now greater than ever before, it is important to recognize that change is never universally acceptable or easy to manage. In spite of the fact that the leaders of the health professions and government are supporting change, there are still logistical barriers to its actual implementation.

Interprofessional issues

Few, if any, of the roles proposed for the community pharmacist are new; they are only new to pharmacy. Thus they are currently being provided by others, and for community pharmacists to develop these roles as their own may be perceived as boundary encroachment by the existing suppliers of the service. Some of the new roles proposed for the community pharmacist, such as a wider role in the treatment of symptoms of minor ailments, which will inevitably result in an element of diagnosis, could also be seen as a focus for further rivalry between professions. Diagnosis is often considered to be solely an activity for the medical profession and any attempt by community pharmacists to participate in this is regarded as encroaching on medical territory (Ashley, 1992).

However, GPs should welcome the contribution that community pharmacy could make to a reduction in their workload, and the improved overall service that is made available to the patient. Nevertheless, the response of the medical profession to an extended role for the community pharmacist has not always been totally supportive, and the pharmacists' ability to provide appropriate advice has been questioned using evidence from the treatment of asthma and childhood diarrhoea respectively (Gibson et al, 1993; Goodburn et al, 1991).

It is inevitable that the extended role of the pharmacist will be seen as a threat by other health care professions, not only by doctors, but also, for example, by nurses, who may be wary of competition for scarce resources. Some of the roles that community pharmacists have traditionally held, such as OTC counselling for minor illnesses, are now being delegated to nurses (Marsh and Dawes, 1995) and nurse practitioners (Lenehan and Watts, 1994) in health centres. Additionally, as noted in Chapter 3, selected nurses now have authority to prescribe a range of drugs. Competition for similar areas of an extended role might therefore seem inevitable, but mutual support and the development of a symbiotic relationship, bringing together traditional clinical and nursing skills, with specialized drug knowledge, must surely be to the greater advantage of both professionals and the public. It is therefore encouraging that, in one study (Bond et al, 1993), community pharmacists supported an NHS prescribing role for the nurse.

Intraprofessional issues

Although professional reports recommending an extended role for the community pharmacist have been endorsed by the RPSGB (*Pharmaceutical Journal,* 1992c), the concept has not received wholehearted support from all members of the profession because of remuneration and commercial pressures. At present, the bulk of remuneration is linked to the dispensing task, although in Scotland, a significant sum is assigned to the payment of a professional allowance, for which the pharmacist has to fulfil key criteria, including dispensing a minimum number of prescriptions, giving advice and displaying health promotion leaflets.

However, the advisory role is still seen by many as using time for which they are not paid directly, and this is a real barrier (Mottram et al, 1995; Savage, 1997). Additional barriers include the commercial environment in which the pharmacist works and the perceived lack of privacy for discussing sensitive topics. At the moment, very few pharmacies have dedicated counselling areas, although most have a quiet area (Bond, 1995). Private areas have been requested by patients (McElnay et al, 1993) and academics (Barber et al, 1994), but they have never been rigorously evaluated.

A further barrier concerns educational requirements. There is a need to continually monitor, and support as necessary, the skill and knowledge base of pharmacists and their assistants to ensure that they can diagnose, communicate and advise appropriately. This is being addressed at undergraduate level through curriculum change, and at post-graduate level through the requirement by the RPSGB for 30 hours of continuing education per year. There has also been investment at a national level with the establishment of the Centre for Pharmacy Postgraduate Education (CPPE) in England, and equivalent organizations in Scotland, Wales and Northern Ireland (*Pharmaceutical Journal*, 1992d). The establishment of the College of Pharmacy Practice has further supported the ethos of ongoing professional development.

The new OTC medicines have accelerated and highlighted the need for the educational changes for the pharmaceutical profession. They have also raised an awareness of the educational needs of pharmacy assistants, for whom, until recently, there were no statutory training requirements. All counter staff involved in the sale of medicines now have to hold an approved qualification (the equivalent of a national vocational qualification, or NVQ, retail certificate test unit 217) (*Pharmaceutical Journal*, 1994b; Evans and Moclair, 1994), which means that all such staff will have a minimal training in identifying correct treatments for specified symptoms and an awareness of those occasions when the pharmacist must be consulted.

Another way of providing relevant training is by the development of clinical guidelines for use in community pharmacies, by both pharmacists and their assistants. These should ideally be produced by multidisciplinary groups and be as far as possible evidence based. One such example is the guideline for the OTC treatment of dyspepsia referred to earlier (Bond, 1994b).

A final barrier relates to pharmacists' liability when taking on new roles from their community base, whether in the high street or the surgery (Appelbe, 1997). All pharmacists are required by their Code of Ethics to have appropriate indemnity arrangements in place, and, if they are in doubt, pharmacists are advised to discuss with the administrators of such schemes the specific tasks they undertake. In the event of a case arising in association with an action shared with the GP, liability would be shared between the two professionals on the basis of case law; in the event of an issue arising from the OTC sale of a medicine, the manufacturer would be liable if the patient suffered an untoward event attributable to the medicine, but the pharmacist could be liable if it were proved that the selling of the medicine was in error.

In spite of all these barriers, there are overriding incentives for the profession to change. By advising the patient and GP face-to-face and using unique skills, the pharmacist can increase the professionalization of the primary care branch of the profession. Individual pharmacists have reported increased job satisfaction when participating in the monitoring and control of repeat prescribing; this might be expected to translate to all new roles. Pharmacists could also indirectly benefit commercially because patients would realize the benefits of buying their self-medication from an informed professional who could advise them and maintain their overall medication record, in contrast to the *ad hoc* purchases of General Sales List (GSL) medicines from other retail outlets.

Patient issues

It is undeniable that the patient has a conflicting perception between the pharmacist as health care professional and as commercial retailer. There are concerns regarding the confidentiality of information, both from the practical aspects of being overheard in the pharmacy and the professional requirement of the pharmacist to respect information. The public are generally reported to be satisfied with the service they receive, but there is evidence that their expectations are not informed by an understanding of the pharmacist's skills, responsibilities and liabilities (Grampian Local Health Council, 1993), and there is a need to market any new services (Williamson et al, 1992). This situation may have been remedied in part by the press release from the RPSGB (*Pharmaceutical Journal*, 1994a) regarding supervision protocols and by campaigns such as National Pharmacy Awareness Week in June 1995 (*Pharmaceutical Journal*, 1995). In order that OTC use of drugs may safely expand, the public themselves will also need to be further educated about the use of medicines, so that they can take on a certain amount of responsibility for themselves. Patients need to accept and expect that community pharmacists will give additional advice and counselling when selling medicines, even if it is not asked for directly. This cannot be seen as an invasion of privacy but as an essential component of non-prescription medicine use, particularly for the more potent P medicines. Many patients feel that they do not want or need advice, for a variety of reasons, such as previous use of the product or advice received elsewhere (Taylor, 1994). If the range of deregulated products increases the number of medicines available from community pharmacies, the public must understand that counselling is an integral part of the acquisition process and, even when that advice is not specifically requested, learn to take advantage of the information offered to them. The public also have to understand that the pharmacist has to ensure that OTC advice and sales are appropriate, and accept the consequent need to ask questions that may appear unnecessary and intrusive. Although the questioning protocols have been criticized (Tully et al, 1997), there is also evidence that if pharmacists and their staff were better trained in communication and the public were educated to understand the purpose, this particular barrier could be readily addressed (Morris et al, 1997).

Conversely, there are incentives for patients to support an extended pharmaceutical role in primary care. By seeking advice in high street premises, they have the support of a trained health care professional with a specialist expertise in drugs, they do not need an appointment, and there is an established network of easily accessible premises. Whilst a private purchase of drugs incurs an additional direct cost, as noted earlier, avoiding a visit to both pharmacist and GP saves on indirect costs; those normally paying the prescription levy may also save on the cost of the drugs themselves.

Future Practice

New models of practice

In their 'high street role', community pharmacists are expected to juggle the roles of dispenser, health-promoter, advice-giver, information-provider for general medical practitioners, and shop manager (Harding and Taylor, 1994), and many opportunities are also open to them (Figure 5.1). As public awareness increases, this juggling will become unmanageable unless tasks are prioritized and some, for example the nominal pharmaceutical supervision of dispensing, as originally proposed in the Nuffield Foundation Report (1986), discarded. Alternative models of delivering pharmaceutical care, such as the merger of pharmacies sharing a population of patients, may need

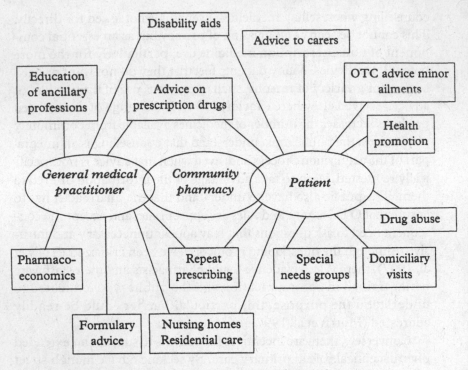

Figure 5.1: Opportunities for the community pharmacist
OTC = over-the-counter.

to be explored. This would enable two pharmacists to share existing professional activity and take on new tasks together (National Audit Office, 1992). Alternatively or additionally, more tasks associated with dispensing and counselling could be delegated to assistants, who would, with increasing training, be able to filter out some enquiries, just as the GP is supported by the nurse/receptionist.

If we consider first retaining the community pharmacists in the traditional high street location, opportunities that could be considered are, for example, multi-partnered pharmacy practices. This would mirror the medical primary care model, in which average practice size is four partners, and single partner practices are extremely rare. This model would allow individual community pharmacists to develop specific areas of expertise and interest, for example analytical and diagnostic processes, domiciliary visits or health promotion, leaving other partners to continue to support traditional core roles such as dispensing and the developing roles at the GP interface, such as prescribing and formularies. For example, one of the partners could feasibly spend regular time at the local surgery, providing direct advice to patients at special clinics such as asthma clinics (Mackie, 1993).

Some community pharmacists already have a dispensing base within a health centre (Bond et al, 1992). These pharmacists tend to have better communication with the local GPs than do the more traditional 'high street' pharmacists. Such pharmacists were said to be 'in a privileged position in that none of their advice need be commercially orientated'(Harding and Taylor, 1990). What is currently proposed is that there are sufficient tasks outside the traditional dispensing role that could fully employ a pharmacist. Some arguments for this have already been published (Ford and Jones, 1995), and the feasibility of such a 'consultant community pharmacist' has already been established and its cost-effectiveness demonstrated (Fogarty, 1995; Hamley and Cromarty, 1995).

The devolution of primary care budgets to fundholding GPs has allowed these types of initiative to be explored and enabled community pharmacists to compete equally with other health care professionals for a place in 'the team'. The possibility of pharmacists becoming partners in general practices could then become a reality, a scenario that would be allowed within current professional codes of ethics, as long as it was a non-dispensing appointment and the prescribing and dispensing roles remained separate. Historically, the prohibition on linking community pharmacists and GPs because of separating the two parts of the prescribing/dispensing process has favoured the development of the pharmaceutical profession, but it has now become a professional liability and is inhibiting links being made that are not centred on the distributive dispensing process.

As 'the costs of providing drugs and appliances to patients constitutes the largest single element of the NHS primary care budget' (Scottish Office Home and Health Department, 1991), it would seem most logical for pharmacists to be central to the management of this practice area. Their acceptance as equal partners would provide the profession with a morale-boosting injection. Partnerships would also further enhance the building of trusting relationships, and even roles such as drug selection for individual patients after initial diagnosis by the GP might become more widely accepted. Such a consultant pharmacist would need to complement rather than threaten the emerging role of the nurse practitioner, who is also seen as contributing to the more efficient use of primary health care services by practising autonomously. At present, it is proposed that this be from within the health centre or medical practice, relieving the GP of the treatment of minor injuries and illnesses and other nurse-oriented tasks, as has already been successfully demonstrated. As GPs' confidence in the ability of pharmacists increases, these roles could be

delivered in the future from a range of locations, including the traditional community pharmacy premises on the 'high street'. As this role
developed further, the frequency of needing to recommend drug
treatment would also increase. A triumvirate of doctor, nurse and
pharmacist could be a very powerful and efficient combination that
could provide a previously unparalleled level of service to patients.

The development of a role for pharmacists within the general
practice base should not obviate the need for 'high street' pharmacies.
It would be an additional model for delivering pharmaceutical care
that would allow the exploitation of a wider range of pharmacists'
skills.

Patient registration

A greater clinical involvement of community pharmacists in primary
care would be facilitated by registration with a pharmacy of the
patient's choice, records being maintained for both prescribed medications and certain OTC medicines (Ford and Jones, 1995).
Records of specific OTC sales are already made in New Zealand
(Macarthur, 1993). This system could strengthen the link between
GPs and pharmacists, provide enhanced continuity of care for the
patient, legitimize the advice to, and monitoring of, patients by the
pharmacist and provide an infrastructure for the delegation of more
therapeutic responsibility (Maguire, 1994). It could be recognized by
remuneration as an incentive to the pharmacist (Jepson and
Strickland-Hodge, 1993). Registration has been successfully introduced in other countries. In America, patients are more likely to be
registered with a single community pharmacy than with a single family physician (Mays, 1994); in Finland, some pharmacies have infor-
mally established a system of 'regular' customers (Lilja, 1994); and
patients are registered with a pharmacy of their choice in the
Netherlands (Department of Health and Royal Pharmaceutical
Society of Great Britain, 1992; Jepson and Strickland-Hodge, 1993).

For the OTC role of the community pharmacist to be fully integrated within the primary health care team, an interchange of information on all medication taken by a patient must be encouraged by
optimizing the potential of information technology (see Chapter 8).
Possible mechanisms would need to be rigorously evaluated. Newer
systems that could be used are 'smart' cards (National Health Service
Management Executive, 1990), which have been piloted, and optical
cards (Beattie, 1995). Community pharmacy, general practice and
secondary care should all be linked for selected information

exchange; this could be done electronically through a modem (Diamond, 1992) or the dedicated NHS information network. For all these proposals, the initial investment is high, and there also needs to be a collaborative and co-ordinated multi-disciplinary approach that would include administration and central funding.

Remuneration

The tying of remuneration largely to the dispensing task, and the expectation of the government that community pharmacists will in part rely on commercial sales to supplement their income, has meant, historically, that any payment for the advisory role is closely tied to the profit on the sale of goods. The pharmacist could therefore be accused of sometimes sacrificing professional judgement in the interest of making a profit on a sale, although there is evidence against this (Cary Market Research, 1994), and many advice contacts in community pharmacy result merely in the provision of free advice (Smith, 1992; Bond, 1995).

Further strengthening of the community pharmacist's role would be provided if it were supported by the NHS. Funding for the NHS prescription of a restricted formulary of products would further develop the OTC advisory role. This might relieve the GP of those consultations in which the main desired outcome, from the patient's perspective, is a prescription for a medicine such as a simple analgesic. Although this may well be currently available from the pharmacy without a prescription, the retail price may be prohibitive for patients who are exempt from NHS prescription charges (Whitehouse and Hodgkin, 1985). Whilst this move would possibly be against the main rationale of the deregulation trend, since it would transfer costs back to the NHS, it would have considerable savings in GP time. Mechanisms, based on means testing, could also be introduced to restrict those eligible for such pharmacy-generated prescriptions. The full economic effect of various options such as these would need to be evaluated.

Similarly, other aspects of the extended role could be remunerated appropriately and individually so that pharmacists would be paid for the specific skills that they would offer, thus allowing professional viability without a dependence on commercially motivated sales. This would be preferable to the professional allowance being further increased, as it would recognize and remunerate individual effort, much as was done with the 1990 contract for GPs (Department of Health, 1989; see also Chapter 2). These innovations would have implications for health care budgets, and the health outcomes and health economic benefits of such an initiative would need to be clearly demonstrated.

Conclusion

As long ago as 1977, the RPSGB gave evidence to the Royal Commission on the NHS proposing that the retail pharmacist's ability to give advice on the treatment of minor ailments be properly recognized and that pharmacists should be able to 'prescribe' certain drugs at present reserved for prescription only. A report commissioned by the RPSGB identified that community pharmacists would like more drugs available to them to counter-prescribe (Hamilton and Dunn, 1985). The pharmacist's involvement in patient counselling at that time was seen to be growing but to be limited unless the powers of the pharmacist were increased. A recent convergence of professional and government agendas has driven forward moves that have fulfilled this proposal. The role of community pharmacy is being extended in parallel with changing patterns of health care. As highlighted in previous chapters, the resources of the NHS are stretched by increased demands and expectations, and there is a perceived need to utilize all resources optimally; the rapid explosion of knowledge means that no one person can remain an autonomous expert, teamwork has to come in the future, and, as a member of the team, the community pharmacist must have a clear responsibility and remit.

It is tempting to conclude that the paradigm of pharmacy is changing concurrently to a more patient-oriented role. Table 5.3 sets the changes of role for hospital and community pharmacy against the parallel development of the medical profession.

There are problems when extending the role of one profession appears to encroach on another profession's boundaries. For such changes to be successful, the mutual benefits must be understood by the 'grass roots' of the professions as well as by the official bodies. There are many new areas of pharmacy practice that GPs would be happy to see introduced; if these can be developed successfully, this might encourage greater interprofessional trust and respect, which would lead to support for the subsequent introduction of the more controversial roles.

An increasing role for the currently under-utilized pharmacist is inevitably and inextricably linked to the greater range of potent drugs available, an understanding of their mechanisms of action,

Table 5.3: The chronological development of the pharmaceutical profession's relationship to the medical profession

Year/decade	Pharmacy role	Medical role	CP skills	Perception	Paradigm	Remuneration
<1840	*Apothecary* Advice-giving Compounding of medicines Provision of medicines	*Surgeons* Treatment				
1841	*Chemist and druggists* Advice-giving on minor ailments Provision of medicines Compounding of medicines Dispensing for doctors	*Physicians* Advice on illness *Surgeons* Treatment	Diagnosis Compounding of galenicals Quality assurance of raw materials	High public esteem High self-esteem Moderate professional esteem	Technically oriented Patient oriented	Market driven Private
1910	*Community pharmacy* Advice-giving on minor ailments Provision of medicines (contd)	*General practitioners* Panel patients Private patients	Diagnosis Compounding of galenicals Quality assurance of raw materials	High public esteem High self-esteem Moderate professional esteem	Increased technical orientation Decreased patient orientation	Market driven Private

(contd)

Table 5.3: (contd)

Year/decade	Pharmacy role	Medical role	CP skills	Perception	Paradigm	Remuneration
1910 (contd)	Compounding of medicines Dispensing for doctors *Hospital pharmacy*	*Hospital physicians and surgeons*				
1948 NHS Act	*Community pharmacy* Dispensing for doctors *Hospital pharmacy* Increased medical knowledge Demand for bulk production Manufacture of parenteral preparations	*General practitioners* NHS patients Private patients Low status *Hospital physicians and surgeons* Greater specialization	No diagnosis Compounding of galenicals Dispensing of tablets Quality assurance of raw materials In hospital, increased manufacturing, quality assurance of raw materials, microbiology	Moderate public esteem Moderate self-esteem Moderate professional esteem	Technically oriented Commercially oriented	Nationalized pharmaceutical service Commercial supplement

(contd)

Table 5.3: (contd)

Year/decade	Pharmacy role	Medical role	CP skills	Perception	Paradigm	Remuneration
1960	*Community pharmacy* Dispensing for doctors	*General practitioners* NHS patients Private patients RCGP (1952) Raising status	No diagnosis Greatly decreased compounding of galenicals Dispensing of pre-manufactured tablets	Decreasing public esteem Low self-esteem Low professional esteem Increasing academic esteem	Technically oriented Commercially oriented	Nationalized pharmaceut-ical service Increased commercial supplement
	Hospital pharmacy Increased medical knowledge Demand for bulk production Manufacture of parenteral preparations Start of ward pharmacy	*Hospital physicians and surgeons* Greater specialization	In hospital, increased manufac-turing, quality assurance of raw materials			
1970	*Community pharmacy* Dispensing for doctors	*General practitioners* NHS patients Private patients RCGP	No diagnosis Little extemporaneous dispensing No quality assurance Dispensing of pre-manufactured tablets	Lowest public esteem Increasing self-esteem in hospitals Decreasing intra-professional esteem Low professional esteem	Technically oriented Commercially oriented	Nationalized pharmaceut-ical service Increased commercial supplement Cost plus contract
	Hospital pharmacy Increased medical knowledge (contd)	Increased status Primary health care team				

(contd)

Table 5.3: (contd)

Year/decade	Pharmacy role	Medical role	CP skills	Perception	Paradigm	Remuneration
1970 (contd)	Demand for bulk production Manufacture of parenteral preparations Supply and distribution Establishment of ward pharmacy	*Hospital physicians and surgeons* Greater specialization Peak in consultant autonomy	In hospital, increased manufacturing Decreasing quality assurance of raw materials Supply and distribution Ward pharmacy	Increasing academic esteem		
1987 Nuffield	*Community pharmacy* Dispensing for doctors CPP *Hospital pharmacy* Increased medical knowledge Decreasing manufacture (contd)	*General practitioners* NHS patients Private patients Higher status Primary health care team established Multi–partner practices Decreased GP– patient relationship	Increasing diagnosis Increasing patient skills Little extemporaneous dispensing No quality assurance Dispensing of pre-manufactured tablets OPs CE/CPP	Increasing pubic esteem Increasing self-esteem in hospitals Decreasing intra-professional esteem Low professional esteem Increasing academic esteem	Patient oriented Drug oriented Technically oriented Commercially oriented	Dispensing fee per item

(contd)

Table 5.3: (contd)

Year/decade	Pharmacy role	Medical role	CP skills	Perception	Paradigm	Remuneration
1987 (contd)	Supply and distribution Ward pharmacy DTC Formularies	*Hospital physicians and surgeons* Greater specialization Cost-effectiveness of treatments highlighted	Change in undergraduate syllabus MSc courses In hospital, decreased manufacturing Decreasing quality assurance of raw materials Supply and distribution Ward pharmacy			
1990 New GP contract New Pharmacy contract NAO reports	*Community pharmacy* Dispensing for doctors CPP, CPPE GP/pharmacist communication Nursing homes Advice on minor ailments PMRs (contd)	NHS patients Higher professional status Decreasing public esteem PHCT established Multi-partner practices Decreased GP–patient relationship	Increased diagnostic skills Increased patient skills Formal requirement for CE Differentiated post-graduate courses Uniprofessional audit	Moderate public esteem Moderate self-esteem Better intraprofessional esteem Better professional esteem Increased academic esteem	Patient oriented Drug oriented Technically oriented Commercially oriented	Professional allowance and dispensing fee

(contd)

Table 5.3: (contd)

Year/decade	Pharmacy role	Medical role	CP skills	Perception	Paradigm	Remuneration
1990 (contd)	*Hospital pharmacy* Formulary advice Prescribing advice Decreasing manufacture Supply and distribution Purchasing contracts Ward pharmacy	Fundholding Cost-effective prescribing *Hospital physicians and surgeons* Decreasing power of hospitals Trust hospitals Administrative change Community care Cost-effectiveness of treatments highlighted	Dispensing of pre-manufactured tablets OPs In hospital, advice on formularies and prescribing Supply, distribution and purchasing Clinical pharmacy	Increased government esteem		
2000 A future vision	*Community pharmacy* GP/pharmacy collaboration and advice Nursing homes Formal advisors on minor ailments (contd)	NHS patients High professional status Increased public esteem PHCT includes community pharmacist Multi-partner practices	Diagnostic skills Treatment skills Patient skills Formal requirement for CE Differentiated post-graduate courses	High public esteem High self-esteem High intra-professional esteem High professional esteem High academic esteem	Drug oriented Patient oriented	Professional allowance

(contd)

Table 5.3: (contd)

Year/decade	Pharmacy role	Medical role	CP skills	Perception	Paradigm	Remuneration
2000 (contd)	Pharmacy prescribing	Decreased GP-patient relationship	Multi-professional audit	High government esteem		
	PMRs	Fundholding	OP dispensing			
	Domiciliary care	Cost-effective prescribing	Postal dispensing			
	Control of repeat prescribing		Public health and health promotion			
	Dispensing for doctors	*Hospital physicians and surgeons*	In hospital, advice on formularies and prescribing			
	CPP, CPPE	Decreasing power of hospitals	Supply, distribution and purchasing			
	Hospital pharmacy	Trust hospitals	Clinical pharmacy			
	Formulary advice	Administrative				
	Prescribing advice	Shared care				
	Consensus treatment	Cost-effectiveness of treatments highlighted				
	Pharmacy protocols					
	Supply and distribution					
	Purchasing contracts					
	Ward pharmacy					

NAO = National Audit Office, CP = community pharmacist; CPP = College of Pharmacy Practice; DTC = Drug and Therapeutics Committee; CE = Continuing Education; OPs = original packs, PMR = patient medication record.

moves to make more drugs available over the counter, the public demand for more knowledge and the government policy of encouraging greater patient autonomy in health care. Thus the prescribing pharmacist will become the focus of the extended profession, consistent with the Nuffield Foundation recommendation (1986) that the core function of the pharmacist is the sale and supply of medicines and ensuring that 'pharmacy is a professional service that promotes and assures rational drug therapy in order to maximize patient benefit and minimize patient risk' (Sogol and Manasse, 1989).

References

Appelbe G E (1997) The pharmacist and new roles. PIA News, p. 4. Birmingham: Pharmacy Insurance Agency.

Ashley J (1992) Pharmacists and the 'D' word. Pharmaceutical Journal 248: 375.

Axon S R (1994) Dispensing doctors – an international perspective. Journal of Social and Administrative Pharmacy 11(3): 106–11.

Barber N, Smith F, Anderson S (1994) Improving quality of health care: the role of pharmacists. Quality in Health Care 3: 153–8.

Beattie J (1995) The Inverurie optical card. Presentation to DURG (UK) meeting, Aberdeen, May 1995.

Bond C M (1994a) Doctor dispensing: no saving. Pharmaceutical Journal 252: 692.

Bond C M (1994b) Guidelines for dyspepsia treatment. Pharmaceutical Journal 252: 228–9.

Bond C M (1995) Prescribing in Community Pharmacy: Barriers and Opportunities. PhD thesis, University of Aberdeen.

Bond C M, Grimshaw J M, Taylor R J, Winfield A J (1998b) The evaluation of clinical guidelines to ensure appropriate 'over-the-counter' advice in community pharmacies. A preliminary study. Journal of Social and Administrative Pharmacy 15(1): 33–9.

Bond C M, Mathieson C, Williams S, Williams P (1998a) Repeat prescribing: an evaluation of the role of community pharmacists in controlling and monitoring. British Journal of General Practice (Submitted).

Bond C M, Sinclair H K, Taylor R J, Williams A, Reid J P, Duffus P (1995) Pharmacists: an untapped resource for general practice. International Journal of Pharmacy Practice 3(2): 85–90.

Bond C M, Sinclair H K, Taylor R J, Winfield A J (1992) Some characteristics of Scottish community pharmacies: How far has Nuffield been implemented? Pharmaceutical Journal 249: R6.

Bond C M, Sinclair H K, Taylor R J, Winfield A J (1993) Community pharmacists' attitudes to the deregulation of medicines and to their extended role. International Journal of Pharmacy Practice 2: 26–30.

Bottomley V (1989) Reported in: POM to P call to meet government's health challenge. Pharmaceutical Journal 243: 728.

Cartwright A, Anderson R (1981) General Practice Revisited. London: Tavistock.

Cary Market Research (1994) OTC Medicines – Maximising the Opportunity. Twickenham: A&M Publishing.

Cotter S M, Barber N D, McKee M (1994) Professionalisation of hospital pharmacy: the role of clinical pharmacy. Journal of Social and Administrative Pharmacy 11(2): 57–66.

Cox I (1993) Reported in: The community pharmacist in the primary health care team. Pharmaceutical Journal 251: 452.

Datamonitor (1992) UK OTC Remedies in 1992. London: Datamonitor.

Department of Health (1987) Promoting Better Health. Cmnd 249. London: HMSO.

Department of Health (1989) General Practice in the National Health Service: The 1990 Contract. London: HMSO.

Department of Health and Royal Pharmaceutical Society of Great Britain (1992) Pharmaceutical Care: The Future for Community Pharmacy. London: Royal Pharmaceutical Society.

Diamond G (1992) The next step in pharmacy computer technology. Pharmaceutical Journal 248: 683.

Drife J O (1993) Deregulating emergency contraception. British Medical Journal 307: 695–6.

Drury M (1988) Teamwork: the way forward. Practice Team 1(1): 3.

Dunnell K (1973) Medicine takers and hoarders. Journal of the Royal College of General Practitioners 23(supplement 2): 2–9.

Eaton G, Webb B (1979) Boundary encroachment: pharmacists in the clinical setting. Sociology of Health and Illness 1(1): 69–89.

Economist (1993) Medicinal madness: Japan's drug industry. Economist 329(7831): 101.

European Community (1992) Directive for Medicines Classification 92/26 EEC.

Evans D, Moclair A (1994) Vocational qualifications for pharmacy support staff. Pharmaceutical Journal 252: 631.

Fogarty M (1995) Give advice to both sides. Pharmacy in Practice 5(7): 315–16.

Ford S, Jones K (1995) Integrating pharmacy fully into the primary care team. British Medical Journal 310: 1620.

General Medical Services Committee (1995) Reported in: More support for OTC emergency contraception. Pharmaceutical Journal 254: 572.

Gibson P, Henry D, Francis L et al (1993) Association between availability on non prescription beta 2 agonist inhalers and under treatment of asthma. British Medical Journal 306: 1514–18.

Goodburn E, Mattosinho S, Mongi P, Waterston A (1991) Management of childhood diarrhoea by pharmacists and parents: is Britain lagging behind the Third World? British Medical Journal 302: 440–3.

Grampian Local Health Council (1993) Health Watch Grampian Project: A Report of a Survey of Community Pharmacy Services. Inverurie: Grampian Local Health Council.

Hamilton D D, Dunn W R (1985) Report submitted to the post graduate education committee of the Royal Pharmaceutical Society of Great

Britain.

Hamley J, Cromarty J (1995) The role of the clinical pharmacist in the GP surgery. Presentation at DURG Regional meeting, Aberdeen, May 1995.

Harding G, Taylor K (1990) Professional relationships between general practitioners and pharmacists in health centres. Journal of the Royal College of General Practitioners 40: 464–6.

Harding G, Taylor K (1994) The symbolism of time. Pharmaceutical Journal 253: 823.

Harris C, Dajda R (1996) The scale of repeat prescribing. British Journal of General Practice 46: 649–53.

Harrison B (1992) Diagnostic testing and screening in community pharmacy: what is going on? Pharmaceutical Journal 249: 226–33.

Hawksworth G (1992) Hands on experience: establishing the service. Pharmaceutical Journal 249: 234.

Jepson M, Strickland-Hodge B (1993) Patients' choice of pharmacy: the importance of patient medication records and patient registration. Pharmaceutical Journal 251: R35.

Jesson J K, Lunec S G, Wilson K A (1997) Role and requirements of pharmacists working in general medical practices. Pharmaceutical Journal 259: R4.

Lancet (1993) OCs o-t-c? Lancet 342: 565–6 (editorial).

Lenehan C, Watts A (1994) Nurse practitioners in primary care: here to stay? British Journal of General Practice 44: 291–2.

Lewis A (1994) Towards 2000: the role for pharmacy in the new NHS. Pharmaceutical Journal 253: 192–4.

Lilja J (1994) Consumer behaviour. International Journal of Pharmacy Practice 3: 192–3.

Macarthur D (1992) Pharmaceutical Pricing in Japan. Dorking: Donald Macarthur.

Macarthur D (1993) OTC Switches – Hope or Hype? Dorking: Donald Macarthur.

McElnay J C, Nicholl A J, Grainger-Rousseau T J (1993) The role of the community pharmacist – a survey of public opinion in Northern Ireland. International Journal of Pharmacy Practice 3: 95–100.

MacIntyre A M, Macgregor S, Malek M, Dunbar J, Hamley J, Cromarty J (1997) New patients presenting to their GP with dyspepsia: does Helicobacter pylori eradication minimise the cost of managing these patients. International Journal of Clinical Practice 51(5): 276–81.

Mackie C (1993) Reported in: Working together: benefits and barriers. Pharmaceutical Journal 251: 127.

Maguire T A (1994) Patient registration is a must. Pharmaceutical Journal 252: 427.

Maguire T A, McElnay J C (1993) Therapeutic drug monitoring in community pharmacy – a feasibility study. International Journal of Pharmacy Practice 2: 168–71.

Marsh G N, Dawes M L (1995) Establishing a minor illness nurse in a busy general practice. British Medical Journal 310: 778–80.

Martin C (1992) Partners in practice: attached, detached, or new recruits. British Medical Journal 305: 348–50.

Matheson C (1998) Illicit drug users views of a good and bad pharmacy service. Journal of Social and Administrative Pharmacy 15(2) 104–12.

Matthews L G (1980) Milestones in Pharmacy. Egham: Merrell Division.

Mays N (1994) Health Services Research in Pharmacy: A Critical Personal Review. Manchester: Pharmacy Practice Research Resource Centre.

Merrison A W (1979) Royal Commission on the National Health Service. Cmnd 7615. London: HMSO.

Morris A L (1980) Interschool relationships in academic health centers. In The Organization and Governance of Academic Health Centers, Vol. 3, p. 180. Washington, DC: Association of Academic Health Centers.

Morris C J, Cantrill J A, Weis M C (1997) Consumer's perceptions of pharmacy protocols. Abstracts from the 3rd Health Services and Pharmacy Practice Conference, School of Pharmacy, University of London, April 1997.

Mottram D R, Jogia P, West P (1995) The community pharmacist's attitudes toward the extended role. Journal of Social and Administrative Pharmacy 12: 12–17.

National Audit Office (1992) Community Pharmacies in England. London: HMSO.

National Audit Office (1993) Repeat Prescribing by General Medical Practitioners in England. Report by the Comptroller and Auditor General. London: HMSO.

National Health Service Management Executive (1990) The Care Card: Evaluation of the Exmouth Project. London: HMSO.

Nuffield Foundation (1986) Pharmacy: A Report to the Nuffield Foundation. London: Nuffield Foundation.

Pharmaceutical Journal (1992a) Royal College of GPs accepts pharmacy report with reservations. Pharmaceutical Journal 249: 305.

Pharmaceutical Journal (1992b) No pipe dream. 248: 305 (editorial).

Pharmaceutical Journal (1992c) Profession welcomes working party report. Pharmaceutical Journal 248: 314.

Pharmaceutical Journal (1992d) New continuing education opportunities for pharmacists. Pharmaceutical Journal 248: 396–7.

Pharmaceutical Journal (1994a) Society issues press release on protocols. Pharmaceutical Journal 251: 127.

Pharmaceutical Journal (1994b) Protocols and staff training to be added to Code of Ethics. Pharmaceutical Journal 252: 124.

Pharmaceutical Journal (1995) President's Pharmacy Week message. Pharmaceutical Journal 253: 794.

Prescription Pricing Authority (1994) Annual Report. Newcastle: PPA.

Proprietary Association of Great Britain (1994) Reported in: OTC medicines market grows. Pharmaceutical Journal 252: 500.

Roddick E, Maclean R, Mckean C, Virden C, Sykes D (1993) Communication with general practitioners. Pharmaceutical Journal 251: 816–19.

Royal College of General Practitioners (1993) Members' Reference Book. London: RCGP: 145–9.

Royal College of General Practitioners (1995) Reported in: RCGP votes for emergency contraception OTC. Pharmaceutical Journal 254: 185.

Royal Pharmaceutical Society of Great Britain (1995) Annual Report. Council of the Royal Pharmaceutical Society of Great Britain. London: Pharmaceutical Press.

Royal Pharmaceutical Society of Great Britain (1996) The New Horizon. A Consultation on the Future of the Profession. London: RPSGB.

Royal Pharmaceutical Society of Great Britain (1997a) Building the Future. A Strategy for a 21st Century Pharmaceutical Service. London: RPSGB.

Royal Pharmaceutical Society of Great Britain (1997b) Prescription Only Medicines Reclassified to Pharmacy Only Medicines. London: RPSGB.

Royal Pharmaceutical Society of Great Britain and the King's Fund (1996) Investing in Evidence-based Practice in Pharmacy. A Summary of the Report Produced by the Pharmacy Practice R&D Task Force (Chair: N Mays). London: Royal Pharmaceutical Society of Great Britain.

Ryan M, Bond C (1994) Dispensing doctors and prescribing pharmacists. Pharmacoeconomics 5(1): 8–17.

Ryan M, Yule B (1988) The Economics of Switching Drugs from Prescription-only to Over-the-counter Availability. Health Economics Research Unit, Discussion Paper No. 02/88. Aberdeen: University of Aberdeen, HERU.

Ryan M, Yule B (1990) Switching drugs from prescription-only to over-the-counter availability: economic benefits in the United Kingdom. Health Policy 16: 233–9.

Savage I (1997) Time for prescription and OTC advice in independent community practice. Pharmaceutical Journal 258: 873.

Scottish Office Department of Health (1997) Primary Care: Agenda for Action. Edinburgh: HMSO.

Scottish Office Home and Health Department (1991) Improving Prescribing in Scotland. Edinburgh: HMSO.

Secretary of State for Health (1996) Primary Care: The Future – Choice and Opportunity. London: HMSO.

Sinclair H S, Bond C M, Lennox A S, Taylor R J, Winfield A J (1998) Reducing smoking in Scotland: a positive contribution from community pharmacy. Tobacco Control 7: 253–61.

Smith F J (1990) The extended role of the community pharmacist: implications for the primary health care team. Journal of Social and Administrative Pharmacy 7: 101–10.

Smith F J (1992) Community pharmacists and health promotion: a study of consultations between pharmacists and clients. Health Promotion International 7(4): 249–55.

Smith M C, Knapp D A (1972) Pharmacy, Drugs, and Medical Care, 3rd Edn. Baltimore: Williams & Wilkins.

Sogol E M, Manasse H R Jr (1989) The pharmacist. In Wertheimer A I, Smith M C (Eds) Pharmacy Practice: Social and Behavioural Aspects. Baltimore: Williams & Wilkins.

Sutters C, Nathan A (1993) The community pharmacist's extended role: GPs, and pharmacists' attitudes towards collaboration. Journal of Social and Administrative Pharmacy 10(2): 70–84.

Takemasa F (1994) The contrasting philospophies of Eastern and Western pharmacy: meeting of the ways. Journal of Social and Administrative Pharmacy 11(3): 121–6.

Taylor J (1994) Reasons consumers do not ask for advice on non-prescription medicines in pharmacies. International Journal of Pharmacy Practice 2: 209–14.

Todd J (1993) The high street health scheme: promoting health in the community pharmacy. Health Education Journal 52(1): 34–6.

Trease G E (1965) In Puynter F N L (Ed.) The Evolution of Pharmacy in Britain. London: Pitman Medical Publishing.

Tully M P, Hassell K, Noyce P R (1997) Advice-giving in community pharmacies in the UK. Journal of Health Service Research and Policy 2(1): 38–50.

Weir L F C, Cromarty L J A, Krska J (1997) Prescribing support from pharmacists to general practitioners in Scotland. Pharmaceutical Journal 259: R27.

Wells D (1992) Cited in: Pharmacist helps doctors cut practice drug costs. Pharmaceutical Journal 248:.699.

Whitehouse C R, Hodgkin P (1985) The management of minor illness by general practitioners. Journal of the Royal College of General Practitioners 35: 581–3.

Williams A, Clarke G, Bond C, Ellerby D, Winfield A (1996) Domiciliary pharmaceutical care for older people – a feasibility study. Pharmaceutical Journal 256: 236–8.

Williamson V K, Winn S, Livingstone C R, Pugh A L G (1992) Public views on an extended role for community pharmacy. International Journal of Pharmacy Practice 1: 223–9.

Zermansky A G (1996) Who controls repeats? British Journal of General Practice 46: 643–7.

Chapter 6
Primary mental health care

Elizabeth Armstrong and André Tylee

Introduction: an old problem in a new setting?

The majority of people with mental illness are cared for within the primary care system. This fact was demonstrated nearly 20 years ago by Goldberg and Huxley (1980), who used a series of levels and filters to describe the ways in which people with mental illness obtain the care they require (Table 6.1). Their model clearly demonstrated that the vast majority of people with mental illness are treated by their GP and are never referred to specialists. It has been estimated that GP consultations for mental illness outnumber psychiatric outpatient consultations by at least 10 to 1 (Jenkins, 1992a).

Moderate to severe depression accounts for about 5% of consultations in general practice, and the Defeat Depression Campaign has suggested that there is likely to be at least one person with mild depression or worse in every GP surgery session (Paykel and Priest, 1992). Clinical studies comparing symptom levels of depression and anxiety in hospital patients with those attending their GP surgery have revealed few differences, refuting the widely held view that general practice patients represent the 'worried well' (Mann, 1992).

Notwithstanding this evidence, there seems to be a common belief that the role of the GP in the care of mentally ill people is new. Whilst members of community mental health teams may find it hard to accept that such a high proportion of the GP's workload is accounted for by mental illness, many GPs, especially in inner cities, complain of an increase in workload, which they ascribe to increased care in the community. In an inner London study that looked at depression in general practice (Armstrong, 1994), some of the GPs involved were

Table 6.1: Mental illness: levels and filters

Level 1 The community
    260–315/1000/year
                                                        First filter
                                                        (Illness behaviour)

Level 2 Total mental morbidity – attenders in primary care
    230/1000/year
                                                        Second filter
                                                        (Ability to detect disorder)

Level 3 Mental disorders identified by doctors
    101.5/1000/year
                                                        Third filter
                                                        (Referral to mental illness services)

Level 4 Total morbidity – mental illness services
    23.5/1000/year
                                                        Fourth filter
                                                        (Admission to psychiatric beds)

Level 5 Psychiatric in-patients
    5.71/1000/year

Source: Freeling and Kendrick (1996). Figure adapted from Goldberg and Huxley (1980). Reproduced by kind permission of Tavistock Publications.

particularly concerned by an apparent increase in the numbers of mentally ill homeless people.

On the average GP list, there are likely to be about 100 patients with major depression and about the same number with symptoms a little below this level, but the number of patients with psychotic illness (who will account for most of those in the community care system) is likely to be relatively small. There is wide variability in this latter figure – between about 4 and 12 (Strathdee and Jenkins, 1996). The difference depends on a number of factors, including GP interest in mental illness, but the most marked differences are between rural areas and the inner cities. In a survey conducted in South West Thames region (Kendrick et al, 1991), those GPs with higher than average numbers of such patients tended to be working in inner London and near large psychiatric hospitals, to have worked in hospital psychiatry posts and to have psychiatrists visiting their practices.

It may not be accurate to ascribe the increase in homeless mentally ill people in the community to mental hospital closure. Craig and Timms (1992) reviewed a number of studies and concluded that the majority of this group were not those who had been discharged as part of planned closure programmes: most had never experienced long periods in hospital. These authors believed that what they called the 'crisis of visibility' was more the result of a long-term failure to provide adequate community services and to the closure of hostels that had previously acted as unofficial asylums for many mentally ill people.

Although they may be small in number, caring for people with psychoses is time-consuming for primary care teams. Nazareth et al (1993) estimated that patients with schizophrenia and those with chronic physical illness consulted their GP with about the same frequency. In comparison with a control group randomly selected from the practice list, frequent attenders were 11 times more likely to be suffering from schizophrenia. These authors also suggested that the care offered to people with schizophrenia was less likely to be structured than that for people with chronic physical illness. In particular, the tendency of these patients to consult with physical health problems may have diverted doctors from the need to review mental state and medication compliance. It is possible that less systematic care leads to increased consultations – and hence the perception of more work. More structured care regimes may also mean that crises can be largely avoided, with benefits to patients, families and doctors (Bridges and Beresford, 1994).

Patients with depression and anxiety are also large consumers of general practice time, and, since much of this morbidity remains hidden, the burden on the GP may not be so obvious as that created by patients suffering from psychoses. It is none the less real. Tylee (1996) reviewed the evidence. Research consistently shows that about 50% of those presenting to the GP with depression are not detected, although this is an average figure that varies widely and depends on many factors, including the interest of the GP. A further 1 in 10 may be recognized at a later consultation, and about half of those not recognized will recover. Many of the remainder will develop a chronic depressive illness, consulting frequently with a variety of complaints (Mann, 1992). A recent European survey of six countries found that patients suffering from major depression made almost three times as many visits to their GP or family doctor as did nonsufferers (Lepine et al, 1997).

There is a pressing need for a valid health economic assessment of selective serotonin re-uptake inhibitors (SSRIs) versus the older tricyclic antidepressants. The tricyclics are effective and cheap. Their side-effects, although unpleasant, are known. The SSRIs are as effective as tricyclics in depression, and their side-effects may be more acceptable to patients, but they are much more expensive than the older drugs. There has recently been a rapid increase in SSRI prescribing (Donaghue et al, 1996). Fears were expressed some time ago that this could lead to a rise in the NHS prescribing budget of over £100 million (Effective Health Care, 1993).

What is primary care?

As noted in Chapter 1, primary health care is the first contact service. It is primary care professionals, most often GPs, to whom people go when they first consider themselves to be in need of help for their health. The average GP has about 1900 patients on his list. GPs do not 'discharge' patients at the end of an episode of illness: any patient may consult again at any time and for any reason. This also applies to other primary care workers, such as practice nurses, whose potential clientele includes anyone on the practice list, and health visitors and district nurses, whose caseloads come from the list of the practice to which they are attached. In inner city areas, where health visitors may work geographically, the caseload will be all families within the area – as well as anyone else requiring health visiting help. The inner city district nurse may also work geographically and relate to several local GPs rather than one practice.

Contact with a GP or practice nurse is generally patient initiated, although patients may attend special clinics, for example the Well Woman clinic, by invitation from the practice. Health visitors usually work more proactively, frequently making the first contact with their clients. District nurses will take most of their referrals from GPs or hospitals. However, not all primary care services are general practice based.

As well as providing the first contact service, primary care professionals, especially nurses, are also engaged in other activities in general practice and the community (see Chapters 3 and 4). They provide a large amount of ongoing care to people with existing illness and disability through chronic disease management clinics (especially for diabetes and asthma), in people's homes and in residential care of various types (Ross and MacKenzie, 1996). The last two of these activities may be described as 'community care' rather than 'primary care'.

The idea of community care has been around for at least 35 years. The large-scale closure of mental hospitals began in the 1960s following the then Minister of Health, Enoch Powell's, Hospital Plan of

1962. According to the 1989 White Paper *Caring for People: Community Care in the Next Decade and Beyond* (Department of Health, 1989), community care means providing the right level of intervention and support to enable people to achieve maximum independence and control over their own lives. This White Paper envisaged a wide range of provision but also recognized that much 'community care' was, in effect, informal care by family members. The National Health Service and Community Care Act 1990 that followed the White Paper set out the responsibilities of health and social services to provide care appropriate to the client's need. This seems to presuppose that clients in need of 'community care' will be those with existing illness and/or disability, whether physical, mental or both. Thus 'community care' is not the same thing as primary care, and community care responsibilities form only part of the work of primary care teams.

Freeling and Kendrick (1996) have placed the tasks of primary care within a preventive framework, here applied to mental health but equally applicable to all aspects of health care:

• *Primary prevention* includes offering support to people at increased risk of mental illness, for example the unemployed, the bereaved, new mothers, single parent families, the isolated elderly and the disabled.
• *Secondary prevention* includes early identification and effective treatment for mental illness. The general practice setting offers a non-stigmatizing environment in which this can happen, but it is also essential that there is rapid and easy access to specialist support when it is required.
• *Tertiary prevention* is about the provision of ongoing care and support for those with chronic illness and persistent disability. In many cases, this will necessitate effective joint working between specialist services, local authority services and the primary health care team. There also needs to be rapid access to help for those whose conditions are likely to relapse or recur.

Primary care professionals and mental illness

Before considering new ways of providing care to patients with mental illness in primary care, it is helpful to look at the differences between primary care and other parts of the NHS that follow from the above. It is also important to understand what is happening now and what the disadvantages of current practice for the mentally ill are.

A key feature of primary care is that practitioners see the whole range of mental illness and distress from mild disorders and problems to severe psychosis. GPs are, in the main, available to members of the public without referral. Everyone is entitled to be registered with a GP, and any person on a GP list may consult that doctor at any time. It is this accessibility and universality which is the main distinguishing feature of primary care.

GPs and other primary care practitioners therefore have to be alert to a wide range of medical problems with which patients may consult. Most secondary care physicians have at least the benefit of a referral letter and are normally working within a defined speciality. The gynaecologist can reasonably assume that all patients referred will be women with a gynaecological problem; the GP has no such advantage. GPs and practice nurses, who are accustomed to being consulted by the patient, may not see themselves as having any proactive role. This may have serious implications for the care of patients with psychotic illness, especially those on depot neuroleptic medication, where failure to attend may be an indication of a worsening of mental state. If such a default is not actively followed up, relapse and then crisis may result. In a survey by Kendrick and colleagues (1991), the majority of GP respondents said they usually only came into contact with people with serious mental illness when a crisis arose in their care. Only 2% of doctors in this survey reported any practice policies for dealing with this group of patients.

Non-psychotic illness

As noted earlier, most of the mental illness dealt with by GPs is non-psychotic illness such as depression and anxiety. In the past, many of these patients may have been referred to community psychiatric nurses. In 1990, community psychiatric nurses were spending as much of their time with this group of patients as they were with people with serious mental illness (Gournay, 1996). This was often believed to be highly cost-effective, but Gournay and Brooking (1995) contend that this belief was based on no good evidence. Their research showed no difference in outcome for patients with depression cared for by either a community psychiatric nurse or a GP. Furthermore, there was no relationship between clinical improvement and the amount of contact the patient had with a community psychiatric nurse, nor did patients seeing a community psychiatric nurse reduce their use of the GP. This has proved a controversial study, especially given the small sample size involved, but the authors believe that there is very little other evidence that community psychiatric nurses are cost-effective in generic rather than specialist roles, although clearly, in pure cost terms, they are cheaper to employ than GPs. A major disadvantage of the use of community psychiatric nurses to treat non-psychotic illness was that it led to a situation in which 80% of patients with schizophrenia did not have access to a trained mental health nurse. According to Goldberg and Gournay (1997), there is evidence that community psychiatric nurses may still be targeting people with non-psychotic illness in primary care, a situation that they attribute at least partly to the employment of community psychiatric nurses by GP fundholders.

All primary care nurses probably have considerable involvement with patients with mental health problems. The high prevalence of depression and anxiety must make it highly unlikely that practice nurses can avoid such involvement; however, in a recent survey conducted for the National Depression Care Training Centre (Armstrong, 1997), only 4% of respondents said that they were involved with people suffering from depression on a daily basis, although just under half had some involvement. In an earlier survey by Thomas and Corney (1992) of practice nurses in two districts, 89% of respondents said that they dealt with mental health problems, and in a national census of practice nurses (Atkin et al, 1993), around 40% said that they were involved in the early detection of depression and anxiety.

District nurse caseloads traditionally include large numbers of elderly people. Depression is more common in older than younger people and the suicide rate higher (especially in males), but there seems to be little published research into district nurse roles in caring for people with depression. Kendrick and Warnes (1997) have reported on an unpublished survey carried out in South London for South Thames West RHA in 1993, which found that district nurses tended to over-diagnose depression and were unable accurately to identify which patients might benefit from extra treatment. These nurses will also be caring for considerable numbers of patients with dementia. The district nurse may be the only professional with whom the carer has contact. Contacts between district nurses, who are usually general-trained nurses and may have little psychiatric experience or training, and community psychiatric nurse colleagues may be limited. The co-ordination of care for people with dementia was a particular concern in the report of the Mental Health Nursing Review

Team (1994), but the role of district nurses was not specifically acknowledged. There are clearly training issues here, but it is unlikely that these will be addressed if the mental health role of this group of nurses continues to be unrecognized.

Health visitors have an important part to play in the recognition and care of mothers with postnatal depression (Cox and Holden, 1994), other mental illness in the post-partum period and mental health problems in families in general. They may also be an important key to prevention. Health visitors are specifically trained in prevention, but the importance of their role in supporting young parents and in teaching parenting skills may not be acknowledged in terms of its potential for preventing mental illness (Newton, 1992).

Psychotic illness

There is much anecdotal evidence, and some research, showing that practice nurses may be quite heavily involved in the care of people with psychotic illness. A South London study has suggested that about two-thirds of all practice nurses in one district may be providing routine depot neuroleptic medication for at least one patient on a regular basis (Garland and Millar, personal communication, 1996). In an audit of patients receiving depot neuroleptic medication conducted in North Yorkshire (Hamilton, 1996), 59% of patients were receiving their injection from a practice nurse. The problem is therefore not confined to London or even to inner cities.

Many practice nurses may also be taking blood tests to monitor lithium levels in patients with bipolar depression. Anecdotal evidence suggests that many nurses regard this as just another task and may be unaware of the needs of these patients.

The national census of practice nurses mentioned above (Atkin et al, 1993) showed that fewer than 2% were qualified mental health nurses (RMNs). Nurses in Garland and Millar's survey (Personal communication, 1996) had little psychiatric training and often felt ill equipped to cope. Further anecdotal evidence suggests that many practice nurses are unaware of the requirements of the current community-based care programme approach (discussed below).

There a number of possible reasons why the latter situation may have arisen. Most practice nurses are general nurses with little knowledge or interest in mental health. They may not see themselves as having a role in mental health care. In addition, it is likely that community mental health teams give them little thought, and since practice nurses, as GP employees, have no management structure and highly variable professional support, there may be no route by which practice nurses can be informed.

Moreover, it is widely acknowledged that depot medication is not popular with patients. Turner (1993) reviewed evidence suggesting that community psychiatric nurses who give these injections may have reduced their other interactions with their patients. Since this seems undesirable, some community psychiatric nurses may have reacted by referring patients to their GP for ongoing medication, leaving themselves free to use other nursing interventions with patients and families. However, it is by no means clear that these other interventions actually happen, and community psychiatric nurses may be depriving themselves of useful opportunities for patient contact.

Although many patients may prefer to receive their medication in the relatively non-stigmatizing setting of their GP surgery, Repper and Brooker (1993) have suggested that many patients in this situation will have no contact with other health service professionals, and their carers may also be isolated. A survey by Murray Parkes et al (1962) showed that only 56% of patients with schizophrenia had maintained contact with their psychiatrist a year after discharge from hospital, but 70% were in contact with their GP. More recently, Meltzer et al (1991) found little change in spite of an increasing emphasis on community care over the intervening 30 years.

To summarize, practice nurses seem to have taken on these tasks almost by default, without the implications being given much thought. Not only may this imply serious problems with the quality of care provided for patients with psychotic illness, but there are also issues of professional accountability for the practice nurse and the community psychiatric nurses (Armstrong, 1995; McFayden et al, 1996). Although nurses are not required to obtain certificates of competence for every new task they undertake, they are nevertheless specifically warned against performing tasks that they are unable to do 'in a safe and skilled manner' (UKCC, 1992a), and they are also warned against the inappropriate delegation of tasks to colleagues without the relevant skills (UKCC, 1992b).

Innovations in care delivery

There is a widespread recognition amongst practitioners and managers of the need for change and improvement in the care of people with mental health problems in community and primary care settings.

A major boost to this movement came following the inclusion of mental illness as one of the five key areas in the Health of the Nation strategy (Department of Health, 1992). Several high-profile cases highlighting failures of care have also helped (see Chapter 4), and, as Strathdee and Jenkins (1996) have acknowledged, many of these failures have been a result of poor communication between various elements of the services.

An important lesson that has been learned is that introducing changes from on high by directive (the 'top-down' approach) is at best a slow and tortuous process, and at worst largely ineffective. One reason for this is that if practitioners are not consulted and do not feel that they 'own' the changes being implemented, they can easily sabotage them. They are, after all, the people who actually provide care for patients, and they are the professionals whose morale will suffer and who may feel threatened if their knowledge and experience are neither acknowledged nor valued. In this section, therefore, we shall consider not only some of the innovations in care that have occurred, but also some of the processes by which change might best be encouraged.

Guidelines

A consensus group has recently reported on an attempt to develop evidence-based guidelines for the care of people with schizophrenia in general practice (Burns and Kendrick, 1997). The group looked at four areas:

1. establishing a register and organizing regular reviews;
2. comprehensive assessment;
3. crisis management;
4. information and advice for patients and carers.

The group acknowledged that there are many areas of practice that have not been carefully researched, and they believed that research into mental health in primary care, although beset with formidable problems, was essential if patients were to receive the care they deserve.

The care programme approach

The basis of care in the community for people with serious mental illness is the care programme approach (CPA), which was introduced in 1991 to provide a framework within which high-quality care could be achieved. From the start, it was intended that its provisions should apply to:

- all people accepted by specialist psychiatric services;
- all psychiatric patients being discharged from hospital.

This was to ensure that no vulnerable person was able to slip through 'the safety net of care' (Department of Health, 1994). It was never the intention that the CPA should apply only to people suffering from psychotic illness, although in some districts it has been interpreted in such a way that only those with a diagnosis of schizophrenia will qualify. Psychiatrists and GPs have expressed concern that an over-concentration on diagnosis as the sole criterion for deciding eligibility for services means that many seriously disabled people with neurotic illness will not receive the care they need. There is a continuing debate about the definition of 'serious mental illness', but it is widely considered that diagnosis is only one of several criteria that should be taken into account. Others include duration and level of disability and also safety and the need for formal or informal care (Department of Health, 1995).

There are four elements to the CPA:

1. systematic assessment of the patient's health and social care needs;
2. a package of care agreed between the patient, the carer, the providers and the patient's GP;
3. the nomination of a key worker for regular contact;
4. regular review and monitoring.

One of the responsibilities of the key worker is to ensure that the patient is registered with a GP, working closely with the primary health care team. Where the patient was initially referred to the specialist services by their GP, this should not present too many difficulties, unless the patient is being discharged to a different area. However, it is undoubtedly working with GPs that causes the most difficulties for community mental health teamss. There may be a number of reasons for this. Community psychiatric nurses may, in fact, have little community training and have moved into community work directly from hospital. It is therefore possible that many community mental health team members give GPs little thought. One published description of the implementation of the CPA in one district says only that care plan summaries and reviews were sent to GPs 'bearing in mind restrictions on the confidentiality of some information' (Shepherd et al, 1995). There is no other mention that GPs were involved in any decision-making at all. Yet it is likely that, at least in some cases, GPs were expected to prescribe for these patients, perhaps depot neuroleptics subsequently administered by practice nurses. There is no mention in this article of this aspect of care other than a very brief reference to treatment compliance.

Many community mental health team members complain that it is impossible to get GPs to attend CPA meetings. Sometimes this is as simple a problem as arranging meetings at inappropriate times. Nine o'clock on a Monday morning may seem perfectly reasonable to most community mental health teams members, yet for most GPs, this is right in the middle of the busiest surgery of the week. This is not a criticism; instead, it reflects an often unacknowledged culture difference between primary and secondary care. It may not be appreciated that general practice is a business. It may be unreasonable, for example, to expect a single-handed GP to attend meetings away from the practice if locum fees are not paid.

Specialist attachments

Before the introduction of the CPA, many community psychiatric nurses were working with primary health care teams on attachment, in much the same way as health visitors and district nurses work. Some of the effects of this have been noted above. Increasing awareness that the community psychiatric nurse, as a specialist, is a scarce and valuable resource and may be best used in the care of the seriously mentally ill (Jenkins, 1992a) led to many community psychiatric nurses being withdrawn from their general practice attachments, often to the dismay of GPs. Ironically, this withdrawal, whilst encouraging community psychiatric nurses to prioritize people with serious illness, may also have adversely affected communication between specialists and primary health care teams. It appears that some community psychiatric nurses are now returning to GP practices, albeit with a much more clearly defined role, which may include acting as key worker for patients of the practice who are subject to the CPA, and being a named link person with the rest of the community mental health team. The link person does not have to be a community psychiatric nurse. Occupational therapists or social workers from specialist mental health teams could also fulfil this role. Key features are a named individual taking responsibility and face-to-face meetings occurring on a regular basis.

There are many more psychiatrists working at least part of the time with primary care teams than in the past, but nationally the situation is highly variable. In a survey undertaken in six health districts in England, Thomas and Corney (1992) found that those practices with links to specialist services tended to have many links, while others had very few. The authors questioned the equity of these arrangements and believed that further research was needed to assess the effect on patient interests. Many GPs welcome input from a psychiatrist, particularly in assessment and perhaps short-term treatment (Strathdee and Kendrick, 1996), but it may be more important to most GPs that, when they refer a patient to a specialist service, the patient is seen by an experienced practitioner rather than a junior clinician who may have less experience than the referring GP (Strathdee and Jenkins, 1996).

Shared care

Diabetes and asthma specialists, and the maternity services, have long been involved in developing shared care systems with primary care teams. Shared care is said to occur when 'the care of the patient is shared between individuals or teams which are part of separate organisations' (Pritchard and Pritchard, 1994). This is clearly the case for those with serious mental illness in the community. A feature of many shared care systems is that record cards are held by the patient. Essex et al (1990) considered that shared care records were acceptable to patients, improving autonomy and communication. Professional and managerial attitudes were the main barrier to further development, but these authors believed that the difficulties could be overcome.

Wolf (1997) also believes that the pooling and simplifying of record systems can reduce duplication and improve communication between services. Moreover, the availability of a patient-held record to all involved in the person's care means that everyone has access to the information they need in order to make sensible decisions, which must involve the patient. Furthermore, this author has reported profound effects on the patients who held their own records. A lady who took her record card with her into respite care took comfort from her file: 'It contained her son's telephone number, and that of her key worker in case she forget them. It provided a link with home and somehow represented order for her.'

Pritchard and Pritchard (1994) believe it to be fundamental that all teams involved in shared care should indeed be teams with common goals and not simply groups of people working from the same building. They have suggested seven steps towards achieving effective shared care, which are listed in Table 6.2. Agreed guidelines, across all teams, are also important, as is the evaluation of the systems that have been set up. Clinical audit is an essential part of this process.

Table 6.2: Seven steps to effective shared care

1. Effective teamwork in all teams
2. Common understanding of the domain – a common language
3. Locally developed and 'owned' guidelines
4. Effective communication and learning – planning should be seen as a learning process
5. Development of alternative pathways for shared care – involve patients
6. Evaluate process and outcome
7. Use audit to refine knowledge base and guidelines

Source: Adapted from Pritchard and Pritchard (1994).

The need for teamworking in mental health care was also a prime conclusion of the facilitator in the Kensington and Chelsea and Westminster FHSA Mental Health Facilitator Project (Armstrong, 1994). Subsequent experience by the present authors in leading practice-based courses in primary mental health care has tended to confirm the view that when teamwork is effective, patient care improves, but research evidence that this is the case is lacking.

The comprehensive community-based approach to mental health care developed in Buckinghamshire and described by Falloon and Fadden (1993) involved working closely with primary care physicians and seems to be the most highly developed form of shared care for mental health so far devised. The authors called their system 'integrated care'. They aimed to provide optimal clinical management for all the people who experienced mental disorders within a defined community. Key elements of the service were:

* early detection;
* intensive interventions designed to:
  – minimize impairment, disability and handicap;
  – minimize the stress suffered by carers;
  – prevent future episodes as far as possible.

Their strategy involved a full range of community services, including primary health care. The focus was on the provision of therapeutic interventions in a natural environment across biomedical, psychological and social management. They found that, with this intensive system, they required minimal mental hospital provision and that specialist day hospitals and out-patient clinics were rarely needed. However, for this approach to work, extensive, ongoing training of the specialist workforce in the latest, cost-effective clinical management was required, together with specific training for primary health care team members, including GPs and community nurses.

The emerging role of generalist community nurses

There has been considerable research in recent years into possible roles for practice nurses in the care of people with depression. McFayden et al (1996) have highlighted the dilemma – whether practice nurses' *de facto* role with seriously mentally ill people should be formalized or whether they should be used to provide care for the much larger numbers of people suffering from non-psychotic disorders who are the mainstay of primary health care. Some may well do both.

There seem to be several ways in which practice nurses can contribute to improving care for people with depression in primary care settings. These include improving detection rates, enhancing treatment compliance, improving patients' access to social support and working with community psychiatric nurse colleagues to improve the access of people with psychoses to health promotion initiatives. Goldberg and Gournay (1997) have also suggested that practice nurses could be trained to use brief interventions with people with phobic and obsession disorders, and also cognitive interventions for depression. If these possibilities are to become reality, there may need to be a huge expansion in the number of practice nurses, and a national retraining programme would be required.

The growth of counselling services in primary care

There has been a huge growth in the provision of counselling services in primary care in recent years. Marsh (1993) believed that this was inevitable given the lack of skill that many doctors have in dealing with those who are 'dis-eased' but not ill in a medical sense. However, as Goldberg and Gournay (1997) have highlighted, there are many problems in defining what counselling is. In addition, the qualifications of counsellors are highly variable, and some may use interventions for which there is no evidence of effectiveness. Most appear to use non-directive methods, which, whilst they may not do any harm to people whose problems may remit anyway, may serve to deprive others of more effective treatment. Corney (1993) noted that some studies suggest that there are some people who may be harmed by counselling. She believes that trials should attempt to identify these groups.

In reviewing the evidence, Roth and Fonagy (1996) have discussed the difficulties of evaluating highly variable treatments with widely diverse patient groups. They conclude that, on the whole, counselling seems most effective for milder illnesses, particularly if specific groups such as patients with bereavement reactions or post-natal depression are targeted. A recent Effective Health Care bulletin (1997) cautions against too wide an extension of counselling services until more is known about the effectiveness of specific interventions and the skills of counsellors.

Facilitation

A variety of primary care projects since the early 1980s have demonstrated the value of facilitation methods in achieving change in primary care practice (Armstrong, 1992). Facilitators work by personal contact to help practices to develop quality care. Important methods include building links between organizations and individuals, and providing education and practical help to enable changes to happen as quickly and painlessly as possible. Practical help might include providing templates and support in designing practice-based clinical guidelines, and in audit of care (Wilson, 1994). Information about services can be disseminated via a facilitator, and feedback can be encouraged. Increasingly, provider units and GP practices are seeing the facilitator role as a crucial element in helping to bring people together and improve the dialogue.

Facilitators may be Trust or health authority employees working on full-time projects. They usually have no clinical role, but most are experienced clinicians. Those currently working in primary care mental health come from a variety of professional backgrounds, the majority being nurses though not necessarily RMNs (Armstrong, unpublished data, 1997). Others may combine a part-time facilitator role with clinical responsibilities. This can work very well provided that there are clear barriers between the two roles and protected time for facilitation activities. Facilitators are agents for change, and it is vital, if change is to be accepted by all stakeholders and implemented, that the facilitator is able to maintain a neutral role, serving the interests of no single person or organization. The purpose is to bring people together so that they can do things for themselves, 'making it easier to understand others and effectively work with others' (Thomas, 1994). If the facilitator is perceived as supporting the agenda of any single group, this purpose will not be achieved.

Meeting needs for training

Earlier sections discussed the degree of involvement that primary care workers have with mental health care. However, such workers, including both doctors and nurses, are generalists who may have little or no formal training in psychiatry beyond that which they will have received in their basic professional education. A survey of GPs in England and Wales (Turton et al, 1995) found that fewer than half of the GPs undergoing vocational training will do a 6-month psychiatry job, although the relevance of such jobs to primary care is debatable. In addition, two-thirds of the GPs had not attended any mental health training in the previous 3 years.

Although many recognize the importance of mental health care for their patients, and may pay some lip-service to concepts of the interdependence of physical and mental health, there may be little attempt in practice to bring these together. It is traditional to eliminate the physical before thinking about the psychological. Jenkins (1992b) considers that it is the specialization in medicine that occurred towards the end of the 19th century which led to the separation of mind and body in medical theory. This has encouraged the 'one patient – one diagnosis' model, which may cause serious disadvantage for those with multiple problems. She believes that doctors miss disease because of a fixation with the 'one diagnosis' model. Psychiatrists miss physical illness, and people with serious mental illness have higher death rates than the general population from common killers such as heart disease and cancer (Department of Health, 1992). Moreover, general physicians, including GPs, miss mental illness, especially emotional disorders (as in the under-detection of depression, mentioned earlier in this chapter). Furthermore, there is evidence to suggest that even people with recognized depression receive suboptimal treatment (Donaghue et al, 1996; Lepine et al, 1997).

These concerns have led to the development of training programmes for GPs in the recognition and management of depression, but there have been some major difficulties with implementing such programmes and encouraging take-up. In Turton et al's survey (1995), respondents considered themselves average or above average at recognizing depression. Why should they think otherwise, unless presented with the results of screening questionnaires? The authors also pointed to a dichotomy between what they term 'perceived competence' and actual competence. Whilst the GPs in the survey expressed confidence in their ability to recognize depression, they felt least confidence in their skills of psychodynamic counselling and stress management. Unsurprisingly, they were most interested in further training in those areas in which they felt least confident. These authors believe that there are challenges here to GP educators in motivating GPs to receive training in an area where research suggests there is a need but where there is lack of awareness of need. There is research demonstrating that appropriate training can lead to improvement in GP performance in both the recognition and management of depression, and also to better patient outcome (Gask, 1992).

In a more recent survey by Kerwick et al (1997) of GPs' mental health training priorities in one inner London area, respondents again put psychological skills high on the list, but psychiatric emergencies was the most frequently selected topic, which is no doubt a reflection of the geographical area in which the study was conducted – an inner city area, where there were likely to be higher than average numbers of patients with serious mental illness.

Community nurse training needs in mental health have been less studied, although a study by Plummer (1995) suggested that practice nurses recognize only about 23% of cases of depression that present to them. There are studies looking at practice nurse-assisted care of patients with depression (e.g. Wilkinson et al, 1993), which showed that nurses were as good as GPs in monitoring patients on antidepressant therapy, and there are studies currently in progress looking at the use of problem-solving techniques with depressed patients. Health visitors trained in fairly basic Rogerian person-centred counselling techniques have been shown to improve the outcome for mothers with postnatal depression (Holden et al, 1989). Much of the research into improving the skills of general nurses in mental health care has been generated by psychiatrists and other non-nurses. It usually involves drafting new skills on to nursing practice, but the skills often derive from disciplines other than nursing and may therefore not fit easily into existing work patterns. There seems to be a widespread perception amongst researchers that practice nurses have more time than GPs. This may not be borne out in practice, and many practice nurses are restricted in the amount of time that their employers will allow them to devote to individual patients.

Conclusion

It seems apparent that the main barrier to improving the care of mentally ill people in primary care is the lack of appropriate knowledge and skills in the workforce. It is important that newly qualified professionals receive training for the job that they will be required to do, and also that the existing workforce has access to appropriate continuing education. This argues for a retraining programme, which, as Goldberg and Gournay (1997) acknowledge, will be massive and will need resourcing.

In the absence of large training budgets, some modest attempts to improve the situation are being made. For example, the RCGP's Unit for Mental Health Education in Primary Care, the College's first teaching unit, has commenced a national Teachers Course in Mental Health Management, which is training district-based doctor/nurse teams to act as facilitators for practice-based education in their own areas (Fogarty, 1997). They could provide an important resource for their health authorities if properly supported in terms of time and money. There are other initiatives in practice-based training, some supported by health authorities but most by the pharmaceutical industry, who, it must be acknowledged, are probably providing the bulk of the currently available funding in mental health education. A Depression Care Training Centre for primary care nurses has recently been established, again with pharmaceutical industry support.

Practice-based training that addresses organizational as well as clinical issues may be more effective in changing practice than the more traditional approaches to GP and nurse education. Speigal et al (1992) suggested that experience in managing change in industry had demonstrated that change happens most readily where there are slack resources. In general practice, there is little spare capacity, so if a member of staff is to take on something new – perhaps a nurse developing a system to monitor patients on antidepressant therapy – something else will have to be given up. Innovations often fail when such practical considerations are discounted.

What is also apparent is an overriding need for the evaluation of team-based training programmes. It is often easier to obtain funding to develop such programmes than it is to evaluate them, but it is vital that good-quality evaluation is carried out. It seems especially important to know whether such programmes really change practice and, furthermore, whether they also lead to improved patient outcome. Future funds will hopefully be targeted to such research, not just for mental health programmes, but also for all aspects of primary health care training.

References

Armstrong E (1992) Facilitators in primary care. International Review of Psychiatry 4: 339–42.

Armstrong E (1994) The Kensington and Chelsea and Westminster Family Health Services Authority Mental Health Facilitator Project: Report of the Project Facilitator. Unpublished report for the Department of Health.

Armstrong E (1995) Mental Health Issues in Primary Care: A Practical Guide. London: Macmillan.

Armstrong E (1997) Do practice nurses want to learn about depression?. Practice Nursing 8(16): 21–6.

Atkin K, Lunt N, Parker G, Hurst M (1993) Nurses Count. A National Census of Practice Nurses. York: University of York, Social Policy Research Unit.

Bridges K, Beresford F (1994) The systematic review in primary care of patients with chronic psychotic illness. Journal of Mental Health 3: 507–12.

Burns T, Kendrick T (1997) The primary care of patients with schizophrenia: a search for good practice. British Journal of General Practice 47: 515–20.

Corney R (1993) Studies of the effectiveness of counselling in general practice. In Corney R, Jenkins R (Eds) Counselling in General Practice. London: Routledge.

Cox J, Holden J (1994) Perinatal Psychiatry: Use and Misuse of the Edinburgh Postnatal Depression Scale. London: Gaskell.

Craig T, Timms P W (1992) Out of the wards and onto the streets? Deinstitutionalisation and homelessness in Britain. Journal of Mental Health 1: 265–75.

Department of Health (1989) Caring for People: Community Care in the Next Decade and Beyond. Cmnd 849. London: HMSO.

Department of Health (1992) Health of the Nation: A Strategy for Health in England. London: HMSO.

Department of Health (1994) The Health of the Nation, Mental Illness Key Area Handbook, 2nd Edn. London: HMSO.

Department of Health (1995) The Health of the Nation: Building Bridges. London: DoH.

Donaghue J, Tylee A, Wildgust H (1996) Cross-sectional database analysis of antidepressant prescribing in general practice in the UK. British Medical Journal 313: 861–2.

Effective Health Care (1993) Bulletin 5. The Treatment of Depression in Primary Care. Leeds: Leeds University, School of Public Health.

Effective Health Care (1997) Mental Health Promotion in High Risk Groups. York: University of York, NHS Centre for Reviews and Dissemination.

Essex B, Doig R, Renshaw J (1990) Pilot study of records of shared care for people with mental illnesses. British Medical Journal 300: 1442–6.

Falloon I, Fadden G (1993) Integrated Mental Health Care. A Comprehensive Community Based Approach. Cambridge: Cambridge University Press.

Fogarty M (1997) Depression training gets a facelift. Medical Interface (April): 38–40.

Freeling P, Kendrick T (1996) Introduction. In Kendrick T, Tylee A, Freeling P (Eds) The Prevention of Mental Illness in Primary Care. Cambridge: Cambridge University Press.

Gask L (1992) Training general practitioners to detect and manage emotional disorders. International Review of Psychiatry 4: 293–300.

Goldberg D, Gournay K (1997) The General Practitioner, the Psychiatrist and the Burden of Mental Health Care. Maudsley Discussion Paper No.1. London: Institute of Psychiatry.

Goldberg D, Huxley P (1980) Mental Illness in the Community. The Pathway to Psychiatric Care. London: Tavistock.

Gournay K (1996) A caring community. Practice Nursing 7(7): 2.

Gournay K, Brooking J (1995) The community psychiatric nurse in primary care: an economic analysis. In Brooker C, White E (Eds) Community Psychiatric Nursing. A Research Perspective, Vol. 3. London: Chapman & Hall.

Hamilton L (1996) Audit of Patients with Schizophrenia on Depot Neuroleptics. York: North Yorkshire Medical Audit Advisory Group.

Holden J M, Sagovsky R, Cox J L (1989) Counselling in a general practice setting: controlled study of health visitor intervention in treatment of postnatal depression. British Medical Journal 298: 223–6.

Jenkins R (1992a) Developments in the primary care of mental illness – a forward look. International Review of Psychiatry 4: 237–42.

Jenkins R (1992b) A multiaxial approach to the primary care of schizophrenia. In Jenkins R, Field V, Young R (Eds) The Primary Care of Schizophrenia. London: HMSO.

Kendrick T, Sibbald B, Burns T, Freeling P (1991) Role of general practitioners in the care of long-term mentally ill patients. British Medical Journal 302: 508–10.

Kendrick T, Warnes T (1997) The demography and mental health of elderly people. In Norman I J, Redfern S J (Eds) Mental Health Care for Elderly People. Edinburgh: Churchill Livingstone.

Kerwick S, Jones R, Mann A, Goldberg D (1997) Mental health care training priorities in general practice. British Journal of General Practice 47: 225–7.

Lepine J P, Gastpar M, Mendlewicz J, Tylee A (1997) Depression in the community: the first pan-European study. DEPRES (Depression Research in European Society). International Journal of Clinical Psychopharmacology 12: 19–29.

McFayden J, Ford K, Rigby P (1996) Schizophrenia and the practice nurse. Practice Nursing 7(13): 21–4.

Mann A (1992) Depression and anxiety in primary care: the epidemiological evidence. In Jenkins R, Newton J, Young R (Eds) The Prevention of Depression and Anxiety. The Role of the Primary Care Team. London: HMSO.

Marsh G N (1993) The counsellor as part of the general practice team. In Corney R, Jenkins R (Eds) Counselling in General Practice. London: Routledge.

Meltzer D, Hale A S, Malik S J, Hogman G A, Wood S (1991) Community care for patients with schizophrenia one year after discharge. British Medical Journal 303: 1023–6.

Mental Health Nursing Review Team (1994) Working in Partnership: a Collaborative Approach to Care. Report of the Mental Health Nursing Review Team. London: HMSO.

Nazareth I, King, M, Haines A, Tai S S, Hall G (1993) Care of schizophrenia in general practice. British Medical Journal 307: 910.

Newton J (1992) Crisis support: utilising resources. In Jenkins R, Newton J, Young R (Eds) The Prevention of Depression and Anxiety: The Role of the Primary Care Team. London: HMSO.

Parkes C Murray, Brown G W, Monck E M (1962) The general practitioner and the schizophrenic patient. British Medical Journal i: 972–6.

Paykel E S, Priest R G (1992) Recognition and management of depression in general practice: consensus statement. British Medical Journal 305: 1198–202.

Plummer S (1995) The Detection of Mental Health Problems by Practice Nurses. MSc dissertation, Institute of Psychiatry, London.

Pritchard P, Pritchard J (1994) Teamwork for Primary and Shared Care. A Practical Workbook. Oxford: Oxford University Press.

Repper J, Brooker C (1993) Valuable insights. Nursing Times 89(25): 28–31.

Ross F, Mackenzie A (1996) Nursing in Primary Health Care. London: Routledge.

Roth A, Fonagy P (1996) Counselling and Primary Care Interventions. In Roth A, Fongay P (Eds) What Works for Whom? A Critical Review of Psychotherapy Research. New York: Guildford Press.

Shepherd G, King C, Tilbury J, Fowler D (1995) Implementing the care programme approach. Journal of Mental Health 4: 261–74.

Speigal N, Murphy E, Kinmoth A L, Ross F, Bain J, Coates R (1992) Managing change in general practice. A step-by-step guide. British Medical Journal 304: 231–4.

Strathdee G, Jenkins R (1996) Purchasing mental health care for primary care. In Thornicroft G, Strathdee G (Eds) Commissioning Mental Health Services. London: HMSO.

Strathdee G, Kendrick T (1996) The regular review of patients with schizophrenia in primary care. In Kendrick T, Tylee A, Freeling P (Eds) The Prevention of Mental Illness in Primary Care. Cambridge: Cambridge University Press.

Thomas P (1994) The Liverpool Primary Health Care Facilitation Project. Liverpool: Liverpool FHSA.

Thomas R V R, Corney R H (1992) The role of the practice nurse in mental health. Journal of Mental Health 2: 65–72.

Turner G (1993) Client/CPN contact during administration of depot medication: implications for practice. In Brooker C, White E (Eds) Community Psychiatric Nursing: A Research Perspective, Vol. 2. London: Chapman & Hall.

Turton P, Tylee A, Kerry S (1995) Mental health training needs in general practice. Primary Care Psychiatry 1: 197–9.

Tylee A (1996) The secondary prevention of depression. In Kendrick T, Tylee A, Freeling P (Eds) The Prevention of Mental Illness in Primary Care. Cambridge: Cambridge University Press.

UKCC (1992a) Code of Professional Conduct for the Nurse, Midwife and Health Visitor. London: UKCC.

UKCC (1992b) Scope of Professional Practice for the Nurse, Midwife and Health Visitor. London: UKCC.

Wilkinson G, Allen P, Marshall E, Walker J, Browne W, Mann A H (1993) The role of the practice nurse in the management of depression in general practice: treatment adherence to antidepressant medication. Psychological Medicine 23: 229–37.

Wilson A (1994) Changing Practices in Primary Care. A Facilitator's Handbook. London: Health Education Authority.

Wolf R (1997) Shared care recording in community care. Nursing Times 93(28): 52–3.

Chapter 7
Service innovations at the primary–secondary care interface: the example of hospital-at-home

Naomi Fulop

Introduction

This chapter uses hospital-at-home as a case study to discuss the issues in the development of service innovations at the interface between primary and secondary care. It begins with a description of the national policy context and some examples of these service innovations, before describing hospital-at-home in more detail. Drawing on the literature and the results of an evaluation of hospital-at-home schemes in West London, the evidence for its effectiveness as a substitute for secondary care is considered. Finally, the barriers to the development of service innovations at the primary–secondary care interface are discussed, and suggestions are made for how the planning of such services should be developed in the future.

The UK policy context

The 1990s have seen the interface between primary and secondary care become a major focus of debate in health policy. As noted in earlier chapters, there have been increasing calls for a shift in care and resources from the secondary to the primary sector (Warner and

Riley 1993; Boufford, 1994; Green and Thorogood, 1998) and the subsequent development of a range of innovations in attempts to achieve this shift. The rationale for these arguments is that health systems with strong primary care services generally have lower costs, higher levels of satisfaction and better health outcomes. Primary care is seen as being able to provide more comprehensive, continuous and holistic care than the secondary sector (Starfield, 1994; Coulter, 1995).

The policy of a 'primary-care led NHS', which began with its focus on the primary care role in the purchasing of services in the form of GP fundholding (National Health Service Executive, 1994), has since developed into a focus on the *provision* of primary health care services (Secretary of State for Health, 1996a, 1996b). Implicit in this policy has been the improvement of primary health care to reduce the need for secondary care services, thereby 'shifting the balance' between the two sectors (Boufford, 1994). A number of different factors have contributed to the development of the focus on this interface, including an ageing population, changes in medical technology, increasing costs and rising consumer expectations (Hughes and Gordon, 1993; Warner and Riley, 1993).

The policy to shift care and resources from secondary to primary care was originally articulated by the Tomlinson Committee, established in response to the effect of the NHS reforms on some of the major teaching hospitals in London. In October 1991, Sir Bernard Tomlinson was appointed as Special Adviser to the Departments of Health and Education on London's health service, medical education and research, with a specific remit to address the provision of health care in inner London within the context of the reformed NHS.

Many of London's teaching hospitals were under threat from competition from each other and from hospitals outside London (for example, in the Shire counties), with purchasers transferring their contracts from the London teaching hospitals to their local hospitals. Tomlinson reported that acute beds in London were over-resourced, whilst primary and community services were underdeveloped (Tomlinson, 1992). A similar analysis had been made earlier the same year by the King's Fund London Commission into the capital's acute services (King's Fund Commission, 1992). Tomlinson recommended the closure or merger of ten inner London hospitals, reducing the number of beds by between 2000 and 7000 by the end of the decade. While attention at the time was focused on these recommendations to rationalize acute services, one of the main arguments of the report was that there was a need for a transfer of resources from the acute to the primary care sector. This argument was based on the assumption that primary and community health services could substitute for acute care.

The Government's response, *Making London Better* (Department of Health, 1993) accepted the broad thrust of Tomlinson and set out its main aim 'to improve primary care for London's population and to pave the way for more cost effective use of London's hospitals' (Department of Health, 1993, p. 5). The London Implementation Group (LIG) was established to oversee the changes, and they in turn set up the London Initiative Zone (LIZ) in inner London to concentrate attention and resources on developing primary care in the inner city. The three objectives of the programme were as follows:

• 'getting the basics right': bringing existing primary care services up to standard (e.g. improving premises and the use of better trained staff);
• developing innovative primary care: supporting initiatives that would bring new forms of primary care to the inner city to meet its special requirements (e.g. the provision of GPs in accident and emergency departments, extended primary care centres, and advocacy services for ethnic minority groups);
• shifting services from hospital to the community: developing the interface between the primary and secondary care sectors so that more care takes place outside hospitals (e.g. hospital-at-home, community beds and minor injuries units).

Both the Tomlinson report and the Government's response assumed that the quality of health care would be improved and costs contained by shifting resources from secondary to primary care (Harris, 1994).

Earmarked monies totalling £210 million made available to LIZ were used for capital initiatives to improve primary care, to improve practice premises and to develop the primary health care team. Resources were also made available on a fixed-term basis to develop revenue initiatives to shift care from the acute sector to primary and community health care. These included hospital-at-home, minor injuries units and GP co-operatives. Similar reviews of acute care were carried out in other major cities throughout the UK, recommending the closure of acute beds and a shift of resources from the acute sector to primary and community health services.

Innovations at the interface between primary and secondary care

In London and throughout the country, acute service rationalizations and attempts to reduce reliance on hospital services have led to the development of a range of innovations that are 'shifting the balance' between secondary and primary care.

While it is not feasible to describe all these innovations in detail, it is possible to give an idea of the range of innovations that have developed. It is important to distinguish between those service developments provided by hospitals which aim to reduce hospital admission or length of stay – such as nurse or GP triage in accident and emergency departments (George et al, 1993; Dale et al, 1995) or hotel wards (Harvey et al, 1993) – and those which increase the proportion of care provided outside hospitals, such as shared care between GPs and hospital specialists. Other innovations involve improvements to primary care that aim to reduce the use of hospital services, such as GP co-operatives (Hallam et al, 1996) and the GP provision of minor surgery (Lowy et al, 1993).

'Shared care' between GPs and hospital specialists is perhaps the longest running innovation at the interface between primary and secondary care. For some years, the majority of pregnant women have received their antenatal care shared between their GP and hospital obstetric department (Bull, 1989). Shared care has also developed for a number of chronic diseases including diabetes (Worth et al, 1990), epilepsy (Taylor et al, 1994), hypertension (McGhee et al, 1994), asthma (Van Damme et al, 1994) and mental illness (King and Nazareth, 1996). These shared care schemes sometimes use a system of shared records between professionals and patients (Essex et al 1990).

Rapid developments in information technology have led to a different type of shift in relationship between secondary and primary care. As discussed further in Chapter 8, e-mail and Internet links have allowed for the sharing of records between GPs and specialists, instant access to laboratory reports (Branger et al, 1995; Petrie et al, 1985) and telemedical consultations (Steele and Wootton, 1997). Although the latter have been in existence for a number of years, they are currently undergoing rapid change and development because of recent improvements in the technology. Video conferences allow for the 'real-time' transmission of a consultation between a GP sitting with a patient and a hospital specialist. These methods can be used for diagnosis and treatment as well as for medical education. Steele and Wootton (1997) argue that there is enormous scope for the development of telemedicine in primary care. There are currently a number of evaluations of video conferencing being carried out in the UK, including a large trial of 'teledermatology'. 'Teleradiology' is being piloted in community hospitals in Aberdeen to reduce patient travel time to distant acute hospitals. Telemedicine is also being used to support nurse practitioners in a minor injuries unit in London with medical advice via a telecare link with Belfast.

Another way in which 'shifting the balance' of care has been attempted is through expanding the range of procedures undertaken by GPs. Encouraged by financial incentives, increasing numbers of GPs are undertaking minor operations in their practices. These include the removal of benign skin tumours, ingrowing toe nails and abscesses (Lowy et al, 1993). Out-of-hours primary care arrangements have also been changing, particularly with the development of GP out-of-hours co-operatives replacing commercial deputizing services. Through co-operatives, groups of GPs work together to provide out-of-hours services for all their patients. This enables GPs to spend less time on call by working within a large rota whilst, at the same time, ensuring that out-of-hours services are provided by more experienced GPs (Salisbury, 1997). These have been encouraged through development funds from health authorities (such as through LIZ in London) and have seen a rapid expansion in number throughout the UK, from around six in 1980 to over 60 by the end of 1995 (Hallam et al, 1996).

GP beds have had a long history, particularly in rural areas where 'cottage hospitals' proliferated in the absence of nearby general acute hospitals. GP beds are in-patient beds that are run by GPs, to which they can directly refer. Although they might be viewed as a shift in the balance between primary and secondary care in the wrong direction – creating more in-patient beds – they have seen a revival in recent years through primary care development funds.

The need for evaluation

The drive to ensure that medical practice is based on research evidence – 'evidence-based medicine' (Sackett and Rosenberg, 1995) – has highlighted the need for health policies, whether at national or local level, to be founded on solid research findings (Ham et al, 1995). A number of commentators have remarked that the policy to shift the balance between secondary and primary care, and subsequent innovations, has either been based on sparse or non-existent evidence, or continues despite evidence to the contrary (Lowy et al, 1993; Coulter, 1995; Scott, 1996; Shepperd and Iliffe, 1996). In a review of the evidence on replacing secondary care with GP-based services, Scott (1996), for example, concludes that the 'cost-effectiveness evidence is scarce and inconclusive'. Furthermore, in an evaluation of the policy to shift minor surgery from secondary care to general practice, Lowy et al (1993) found not only a lack of evidence that this had reduced hospital activity, but also that overall minor surgical activity had increased, suggesting that new patients had come forward for treatment.

These examples illustrate the lack of research into this major policy initiative and the innovations that have developed in its wake. The NHS Research and Development Programme recognized this by establishing in 1994 a national programme in the area of the primary–secondary care interface. There have been two calls for research proposals, and 69 research projects have been commissioned, including evaluations of hospital-at-home schemes, GP beds/community hospitals, GP co-operatives and telemedicine (National Health Service Executive, 1997).

Research in this area, like other health services and policy research (Black, 1997), needs to draw on a number of different disciplines and methods in order to address the range of questions raised. These include economics, sociology, epidemiology, statistics, policy analysis and organizational theory.

Hospital-at-home: a brief history of its development in the UK

In the 19th century and early part of the 20th century, hospitals were viewed as a place of last resort for medical care. However, improvements in drug therapies and anaesthetic techniques, changes in technology and increasing specialization all contributed to the development of the hospital in the 20th century as the centre of the health system. Care began to move out of the home and into cottage hospitals, and, in their turn, cottage hospitals were closed or merged into district general hospitals, relatively large establishments offering care for a wide range of medical and surgical needs, with increasingly specialist staff.

The shift towards hospital care inevitably placed increasing pressure on a system in which supply has been unable to keep pace with demand. Although lengths of stay in hospital have decreased over the past 30 years, the pressure on hospital beds has not declined. In addition, evidence suggesting that there are high numbers of inappropriately filled hospital beds (Victor et al, 1993), and the high incidence of hospital-acquired infection (Currie and Maynard, 1989), has contributed to the debate about the role and development of the hospital in the context of the broader health care system, and has precipitated a search for acceptable alternatives (Coast et al, 1996). In recent times, improvements in housing, the availability of nursing and domiciliary care in the community, the assumption of increasing patient preference to be treated at home, and improved technologies allowing care to take place outside the hospital have made shifting care from hospital to home a much more potentially viable and desirable option (King's Fund Centre, 1989; Marks, 1991).

Although hospital-at-home was well established in other countries, including France, the USA and New Zealand, the first hospital-at-home scheme in the UK was not established until 1978, in Peterborough (Mowat and Morgan, 1982). Although it had a small number of patients in its first year (51 referrals and 32 admissions), the Peterborough scheme has grown to be Britain's largest hospital-at-home scheme, with both an early discharge and a prevention of admission component. Hospital-at-home began to develop beyond Peterborough during the 1980s.

What is hospital-at-home?

Hospital-at-home provides care in the patient's home that would otherwise have been provided in hospital. In other words, if the patient were not receiving care from hospital-at-home, she would be receiving care in an acute unit. As noted earlier, this notion of substitution is important within the context of the Tomlinson report (Tomlinson, 1992), in which schemes were explicitly expected to replace hospital care rather than to provide an extension of hospital or social care. Hospital-at-home schemes in this context had to result in cost savings in the secondary sector so that they could be funded from these savings once pump-priming monies ended. Hospital-at-home schemes in other contexts may have aims in addition to, or other than, the substitution of hospital care.

Hospital-at-home schemes provide care for a range of age groups and conditions. Broadly speaking, there are four types of hospital-at-home scheme (Marks, 1991):

1. Early discharge. The patient is discharged from hospital (for example, following orthopaedic surgery) to his home and continues to receive care from hospital-at-home staff (nursing and therapy). In this case, hospital-at-home usually replaces the later days

of the patient episode, when the need for intensive nursing and medical care has passed.

2. Prevention of admission or admission avoidance. The patient is referred from the community (usually by a GP or district nurse) to a hospital-at-home scheme instead of to hospital for, for example, a chest infection. In this case, hospital-at-home replaces the whole episode of care (unless the patient's condition worsens, requiring more intensive in-patient care).

3. Terminal or palliative care services (often called hospice-at-home).

4. High-tech home care, in which treatments previously offered in hospital (such as dialysis and intravenous antibiotics) have been adapted to be available at home. This form of care is particularly well established in the USA (Shepperd and Iliffe, 1996).

As a result of the policy to transfer care and resources from secondary to primary care, and because of the growing pressures on acute beds, hospital-at-home has become a popular option. A national survey of health authorities indicated that most were either supporting or planning to support a hospital-at-home scheme (Iliffe, 1997). There are a wide range of schemes described in the literature. Some schemes are for patients with specific conditions, such as home ventilation for asthma patients, while others provide specialist services such as the administration of intravenous antibiotics. Other schemes care for a much broader range of conditions, such as one in Gloucester that cares for medical patients (Donald et al, 1995), and 'home-from-hospital' schemes that aim to assist the discharge of frail older patients to their homes, thereby reducing the number of 'bed blockers' (i.e. patients occupying hospital beds when they no longer require acute care) (Waddington and Henwood, 1996).

The most common schemes, however, are those which care for patients following surgery, particularly orthopaedic surgery. Orthopaedic schemes are of particular interest because of both the increasing incidence in hip fracture, resulting in part from the ageing of the population, and a corresponding increase in cost and pressure on resources (Hollingworth et al, 1995). An Audit Commission (1995) report into rehabilitation following hip fracture noted that all of the hospitals they visited that did not have an early discharge scheme were considering establishing one. Schemes for orthopaedic patients were established in Southern Derbyshire in 1990 (Roberts, 1992; O'Caithan, 1994), West London in 1993 (Fulop et al, 1997),

Merton and Sutton in 1993 (Brooks, 1996), Wandsworth in 1995
(Rink et al, 1998) and Kingston in 1994 (Elliot, 1995), among
others.

The development of hospital-at-home in London

The development of hospital-at-home schemes was considered to be
an appropriate use of the LIZ pump-priming revenue funding
described above. Hospital-at-home was almost universally viewed as
'a good thing', a way both to improve care for patients and, many
believed, to shift care and resources from the hospital to the community. It was speculated that hospital-at-home could reduce the use of
acute beds by 50% (Moss and McNicol, 1993).

The development of hospital-at-home schemes and other primary
care initiatives in London offers important lessons. Resources from
the LIG were made available very quickly in 1993, requiring some
health authorities to plan the expenditure of £5–10 million overnight.
Providers were asked to bid for funds but had only days in which to
develop proposals (Snell, 1995). Through no fault of either the
health authorities or the providers, the process tended to be supply
led and based on what providers were interested in rather than decided
on the basis of needs assessment or feasibility studies.

An analysis of the overall LIZ programme by Mays et al (1997)
found that, in terms of funding, by 1995/96, 46% of the expenditure
had gone on premises development, 16% on extending primary care
or widening access and only 16% on shifting the balance of services
between primary and secondary care. In this latter category, the most
popular types of innovation have been hospital-at-home and home-
based care. According to Mays et al (1997), there were, by 1995/96,
20 early discharge hospital-at-home schemes and seven admission
avoidance schemes receiving LIZ funding.

A broad range of hospital-at-home models has been established in
London, including prevention of admission and early discharge
schemes. Paediatric home care teams have also been established
under the rubric of hospital-at-home. A range of organizational models exist, and schemes are managed either by community or acute
Trusts, or by integrated acute and community providers.

The emphasis on evidence-based commissioning (whereby health
authorities and GP fundholders are encouraged to base their purchasing decisions on research evidence) has been particularly strong

for initiatives funded through LIZ, hence the need for evaluation. These schemes have been funded for a limited time, usually 3 years, and health authorities then have to decide whether or not to continue funding from mainstream budgets at the expense of other services. It was originally envisaged that these schemes would be funded from savings on acute care expenditure.

Hospital-at-home – a substitute for hospital?

Given this situation, the key question that needs to be addressed about hospital-at-home is whether it results in the shift of care and resources from secondary to primary care. In other words, can it substitute for secondary care?

The term 'substitution' has been defined as 'the continual regrouping of resources across and within care settings, to exploit the best and least costly solutions in the face of changing needs and demands' (World Health Organisation, 1996). In other words, health care professionals, skills, equipment, information and facilities can be reorganized to achieve better clinical, financial and patient-related outcomes. New technologies in the health sector are continually being substituted for old ones. These may include not only new drugs and surgical procedures, but also new patterns of the organization of health care. Warner (1996) has developed a typology that differentiates between three types of substitution:

- moving the location at which care is given (e.g. from secondary hospitals to tertiary hospitals);
- introducing new technologies (e.g. minimal access surgery);
- changing the mix of staff and skills (e.g. practice nurses for GPs; see Chapter 3).

Some methods of substitution involve a combination of two or more of these types. For example, 'high-tech' hospital-at-home, mentioned above, involves all three types of substitution. The hospital-at-home schemes described in this chapter mostly involve two types: a change in location (from hospital to home) and in the mix of staff and skills (hospital nurses and doctors to community nurses/GPs).

For health authorities in London and elsewhere, where the aim of hospital-at-home was to substitute for acute in-patient care, the 'bottom line' was that hospital-at-home had to show that it could provide care of at least the same level of quality as hospitals, for the same or less cost. Furthermore, if in the longer term, hospital-at-home was to be funded out of savings made in the acute sector, hospital-at-home had to result in significant reductions in acute services (e.g. the closure of wards and even whole hospitals).

Evaluations of hospital-at-home in London and elsewhere have addressed the following questions, which constitute the different elements of substitution:

- How do hospital-at-home costs compare with those of standard hospital care?
- How do lengths of stay compare?
- Does hospital-at-home provide a quality of care better than or equal to that of standard hospital care?
- What do patients think of hospital-at-home, and what are the views of health care professionals and managers?

The rest of this chapter uses results from an evaluation of hospital-at-home in London together with other research findings to address these questions.

Evidence for hospital-at-home

To date, there has been relatively little rigorous research into hospital-at-home schemes in Britain (Shepperd and Iliffe, 1996). Hospital-at-home evaluations (both completed and currently underway) encompass a variety of designs. Until recently, randomized controlled trials have had limited success: two studies that initially intended to conduct a randomized controlled trial found that this was not feasible (Knowelden et al, 1991; O'Caithan, 1994), and one that did conduct a randomized controlled trial found that the method of selection that they had chosen to maximize scheme usage resulted in patients who were not wholly suitable being treated by hospital-at-home (Donald et al, 1995). Other evaluations have used non-randomized comparative designs and non-comparative descriptive studies. However, three randomized controlled trials have recently been conducted in Leicester (Wilson et al, 1997), Bristol (Richards et al, 1998; Coast et al, 1998) and Corby (Shepperd et al, 1998a; Shepperd et al, 1998b).

The four main dimensions along which hospital-at-home schemes have generally been evaluated – patient outcomes (including both physical and emotional health), length of stay, costs and satisfaction (of patients, carers, and health professionals) – are discussed below with reference to an evaluation of hospital-at-home in West London and to other studies of hospital-at-home.

The West London study

The study of hospital-at-home in West London covered five schemes funded by LIZ monies and provided by three health authorities. All five were run by community Trusts; three were early discharge schemes and two prevention of admission schemes. As Table 7.1 shows, they varied considerably in size, the early discharge schemes were more successful at recruiting patients than the prevention of admission schemes. The majority of patients in the early discharge schemes were orthopaedic patients discharged after elective total hip or total knee replacement, or after emergency admission following a fractured neck of femur. The majority of patients in all schemes were women aged over 65 years.

There were three elements to the evaluation. In the first part of the study, a number of process measures, including activity, lengths of stay, management and development of the scheme, were monitored for all the schemes. The second component measured a range of outcomes including re-admissions, clinical outcomes, and patient, carer and staff satisfaction for the three early discharge schemes; hospital-at-home patients were compared with a group of patients who received standard hospital care. Third, a costings analysis of the three early discharge schemes was conducted to see how the costs of hospital-at-home compared with those of standard hospital care (Hensher et al, 1996).

Table 7.1: Total number of admissions during calendar year 1995 and percentage over 65 and percentage female

Scheme	No. of admissions	% over 65 years	% female
Early discharge			
Scheme 1	377	71.1	67.6
Scheme 2	362	56.4	55.0
Scheme 3	154	77.8	72.7
Prevention of admission			
Scheme 4	20	85.0	70.0
Scheme 5	56	46.4	69.6
Total	969	65.4	63.8

Patient outcomes

Marks (1991) discusses a number of studies that have shown that, for certain conditions, hospital-at-home care has the same level of clinical effectiveness as standard hospital care. However, it is important to note that some of these studies are two decades old, and Shepperd and Iliffe (1996) argue that changes in clinical practice and reduced length of stay may make some of these findings redundant in the current health service.

More recently, hospital-at-home has been shown to be as clinically effective for hip fractures (Pryor and Williams, 1989) and elderly medical patients, at least in terms of mobility (Byers and Parker, 1992). Several evaluations have examined the change in functional and quality of life outcomes for both hospital-at-home and standard hospital care patients. One study found that hospital-at-home patients had better emotional health after discharge than did standard hospital care patients (O'Caithan, 1994), but otherwise there are no studies reporting a difference in patient outcomes.

A systematic review of five randomized controlled trials of hospital-at-home found no differences in patient health outcomes, although all the studies were small and lacked power (Shepperd and Iliffe, 1997). Early results from the randomized controlled trials in Leicester and Bristol indicate that outcomes (as measured by mortality, functional status and quality of life) for hospital-at-home patients did not differ from those for patients receiving standard hospital care (Wilson et al, 1997; Richards et al, 1998). The RCT in Corby found few differences in outcomes at three months follow up as measured by mortality, general health status, physical functioning and hospital readmission (Shepperd et al, 1998). Similarly, neither the study of hospital-at-home in West London (Hood et al, 1997) nor that in Wandsworth (Rink et al, 1998) found any overall differences in patient outcomes, as measured by functional status and quality of life. From the evidence available, it appears that hospital-at-home can provide care of equal quality, in terms of patient outcome, to that of standard hospital care.

Length of stay

Length of stay is important because it provides a benchmark by which standard hospital care and hospital-at-home can be compared and therefore costed (see below). Evidence on length of stay is mixed and, in some cases, very unclear. For early discharge schemes, hospital-at-home aims to replace in-patient days with at-home days. Therefore the following total lengths of stay should be compared:

- hospital-at-home: from entry to hospital to discharge from hospital-at-home;
- standard hospital care: from entry to hospital to discharge from hospital.

This comparison was made in the Southern Derbyshire evaluation, which found that fractured neck of femur patients had the same overall length of stay in hospital-at-home as in standard hospital care (O'Caithan, 1994). The evaluation of the Peterborough hospital-at-home scheme found that lengths of stay were shorter in hospital-at-home for cancer, stroke and post-operative care (Knowelden et al, 1991). It is not clear whether this difference was significant.

However, other published results compare the in-patient days of hospital-at-home with those of standard hospital patients (Parker et al, 1991; Donald et al, 1995). This information is useful in terms of understanding the point at which hospital-at-home patients are discharged but does not allow a comparison of overall length of stay, as saved in-patient days are replaced by days at home.

In the West London study, data on length of stay were compared for elective orthopaedic patients for two of the schemes. In both schemes, the total length of stay for hospital-at-home patients was greater than for standard hospital care, but this difference was significant for only one scheme (Hood et al, 1997). These results suggest that, in West London, hospital-at-home is providing a service additional to that of hospital care.

Costs

An important factor underlying attempts to redress the balance between secondary and primary care is the assumption that services provided in a primary or community health care setting are cheaper than those provided in hospital. As discussed earlier, there is little evidence to support this. On the contrary, evidence suggests that, in the specific case of services provided by GPs, these services have become additional to, rather than replacements for, hospital services (Lowy et al, 1993).

In any discussion on costs, it is important to clarify which costs are being measured. Some studies have investigated costs to the NHS (and social services), while others have also considered costs to patients and carers. Some argue that shifting care and resources from secondary to primary care, for example by providing care in the home, shifts the burden of care (and costs) to patients and carers (Clarke, 1996).

The evidence on hospital-at-home costs is mixed. A study of the Peterborough scheme by Hollingworth et al (1993) found that the costs of hip fracture patients discharged to hospital-at-home were less than for patients who received standard in-patient care. A sensitivity analysis showed that this was true even if in-patient costs were 50% lower than predicted or hospital-at-home costs were 50% higher than predicted. An earlier study of the Peterborough scheme included a cost component, with the capital cost of the hospital excluded from the analysis. This study found that costs per day were the same in hospital-at-home and standard hospital care for cancer and stroke patients, and were lower for post-operative care. Shorter lengths of stay meant that overall costs for hospital-at-home were lower, but the authors acknowledge that, for the scheme to make an impact on hospital costs, the scale of its activity would need to be much higher (Knowelden et al, 1991): more throughput was needed.

Other evaluations have included a cost component, but methods of collection and reporting have varied widely. The Southern Derbyshire evaluation compared the price charged by providers of hospital-at-home and standard hospital care. As the author has noted, the price charged for a service is not the same as how much a service costs (O'Caithan, 1994). For example, a provider may have artificially reduced the price of a service by cross-subsidizing it from elsewhere, so this is not a satisfactory approach.

The West London study provides data suggesting that hospital-at-home is more expensive per episode of care compared with standard hospital care. In terms of costs per day, hospital-at-home was slightly cheaper in two of the schemes compared with hospital care; in the third scheme, it was more expensive. However, as discussed above, the lengths of stay for the whole episode were greater for hospital-at-home compared with standard hospital care, thereby making hospital-at-home more expensive per episode of care. The Corby RCT found no difference in total health care costs between hospital-at-home and hospital care for patients with hip or knee replacements or general medical patients; costs for hysterectomy patients and those with chronic obstructive airways disease were higher for hospital-at-home patients (Shepperd et al, 1998b). However, results from the randomized controlled trials in Bristol indicate that hospital-at-home costs to the NHS are lower than those for standard hospital care patients (Coast et al, 1998). It is unclear whether the differences between the findings from different studies are a result of artefact (for example, different methods of measuring costs) or because of the organization of the schemes. It is hoped that when more results from the trials are available, this will become clearer.

The West London study raises the issue of the difficulty of substituting for in-patient acute care because of the fixed costs of hospitals (Hensher et al, 1996). Even if the hospital-at-home schemes had been able to operate at much lower costs (by operating at much higher activity levels), it is doubtful whether, in the long term, they could have been funded out of savings in the acute sector. In order to start releasing resources through, for example, closing a ward, the number of patients treated by hospital-at-home would need to be considerably higher. Even if this were possible and a ward could be closed, the fixed costs of central hospital services (pathology, radiology, etc.) would be spread over fewer episodes of care, thereby increasing the cost per case.

Patients' views

Another assumption that has shaped the policy to shift services is that patients prefer to be treated in the primary care sector, either at home or in local primary health care centres closer to their homes. Again, there is little evidence for this (Scott, 1996). In fact, there is evidence that patients' expectations of being referred for specialist care are increasing (Coulter, 1995).

Studies of patients' views of hospital-at-home are important, then, to see if the assumption holds true. One indicator of this is the number of patients who refuse to be discharged into hospital-at-home schemes but choose instead to remain in hospital. The West London study found that just under 15% of patients referred to hospital-at-home schemes refused to be discharged to them. A small but important minority of patients are concerned about being cared for at home, the main reasons given being that they either did not want to, or perceived that they could not rely on health care staff coming into their home.

Another way to gauge patient views is to compare satisfaction levels between hospital-at-home and standard hospital care. The study of hospital-at-home in Peterborough found that patients in hospital were more likely to express dissatisfaction with their care than were those at home (Knowelden et al, 1991). Early results from the randomized controlled trials in Bristol and Leicester indicate contrasting results. In Bristol, researchers found no significant differences in satisfaction between hospital-at-home and standard hospital care (Richards et al, 1998), whereas in the Leicester trial, researchers found that satisfaction with hospital-at-home was significantly higher than with standard hospital care (Wilson et al, 1997). The systematic review of hospital-at-home found that patients discharged early from hospital to hospital-at-home following elective surgery expressed greater satisfaction than those who remained in hospital (Shepperd and Iliffe, 1997).

In the West London study, there were no differences in overall satisfaction between hospital-at-home and standard hospital care patients – both groups showed high levels of satisfaction. The vast majority of hospital-at-home patients said that they would choose to use the scheme again, and just under half of standard hospital care patients said that they would be interested in hospital-at-home if it were offered to them. However, standard hospital care patients were significantly more likely to feel involved in decisions about their treatment and care in hospital, and significantly more likely to feel ready to be discharged from hospital.

Given the high rates of satisfaction found for both models of care, it seems that, on the whole, patients like what they know, or at least that is what they report in written questionnaires. The randomized controlled trial of hospital-at-home in Leicester found that these elderly patients' recall of experiences was affected by poor memory, confusion and a reluctance to express negative views. Despite expressing dissatisfaction during discussion, the same patient would record a positive view on the questionnaire (Parker, personal communication, 1997).

Views of health care professionals and managers

If the policy to move care and resources from secondary to primary care is to be successful, it is vital that the wide range of health care professionals and managers working in both sectors and at their interface support its objectives. Fears have been expressed that attempts to alter the balance will result in an increased workload for primary and community health care staff, without the additional necessary resources. These concerns have been most strongly articulated by GPs (Husain, 1996). A recent systematic review of the literature, however, found little evidence of whether a shift of services from secondary to primary care results in an increased workload for GPs and concluded that GPs' claims of an increased workload are based on anecdotal evidence (Pedersen and Leese, 1997).

Few published studies have considered the views of health care professionals and managers concerned with hospital-at-home. Studies of the Peterborough hospital-at-home scheme have considered professional issues, describing how hospital-at-home staff were initially organized separately from other community nurses. This caused a number of difficulties: liaison with GPs was problematic; some resentment was felt by existing community nurses; and patients experienced a lack of continuity of care, seeing up to six different members of staff. As a result, the scheme was reorganized and incorporated into the primary health care team (Anand and Pryor, 1982; Mowat and Morgan, 1982; Knowelden et al, 1991).

The study of hospital-at-home schemes in West London included interviews with purchaser and provider managers (including nurse managers) and hospital clinicians to obtain their views. GPs' views were elicited through a questionnaire survey. The main achievements and problems with the hospital-at-home schemes cited in the 19 interviews with managers and professionals are summarized in Table 7.2.

It is important to note that these are the perceptions of these respondents. Although they are sometimes in accordance with the study findings – for example, that hospital-at-home reduces patients' length of stay in hospital – in other cases they conflict, for example in the view that hospital-at-home increases patient satisfaction (the study finding that satisfaction levels were the same for hospital-at-home and standard hospital care). The interview data often confirmed the problems with LIZ-funded projects in general. Managers and professionals were critical of how the schemes were developed too quickly, with no time for feasibility studies or needs assessments to be undertaken. The schemes were not given enough 'start-up' time to recruit staff, build relationships with acute and community staff, and begin admitting patients. Respondents felt that these difficulties adversely affected the development of the schemes. The lack of preparation time is illustrated by the finding

Table 7.2: Main achievements and problems of hospital-at-home

Main achievements	Main problems
Reduced length of hospital stay	Resistance from acute Trusts
Increased throughput on orthopaedic wards	Resistance from GPs and some district nurses
Reduced orthopaedic waiting list	Short start-up time
Contributed to reduction in number of beds	poor management of schemes
	Type of funding problematic
Created more available beds	Difficulty finding enough patients
Improved patient care	Lack of integration of hospital-at-home
Improved quality of discharge	with other services
Higher patient and carer satisfaction	Evaluation taking place too soon
	Leaves higher-dependency patients in
More patient choice	hospital

that although managers and professionals generally agreed that the main aim of hospital-at-home was to reduce the length of stay in hospital, two of the schemes did not have clear performance targets for length of stay written into their contracts.

The interviews illustrate the resistance to hospital-at-home from managers and professionals both inside and outside hospitals. Hospital staff raised concerns about the hospital-at-home schemes recruiting low-dependency patients, leaving hospitals with high-dependency patients (and thus increasing costs for the hospital). One explanation for the low number of admissions to one of the hospital-at-home schemes in West London was the poor relationship between the community trust running the scheme and the hospital from which it recruited its patients. It is interesting that, of the three early discharge schemes, it had the lowest number of admissions (see Table 7.1, scheme 3, above). In one of the prevention of admission schemes, the district nurses were reluctant to take on the extra workload demanded by hospital-at-home patients (Fulop et al, 1997). Resistance was also found from managers in health authorities with responsibility for purchasing acute services who were concerned at the implications of negotiating cuts in the budgets of the acute hospitals with whom they negotiated contracts. A study of hospital-at-home in South London also identified resistance to change among the staff interviewed (Sims et al, 1997).

Given that GPs are medically responsible for patients in hospital-at-home schemes, it is important that their views are also taken into account. In the West London study, 141 out of 183 GPs in two health authorities where hospital-at-home schemes operated responded (a 77% response rate) to a questionnaire survey (Hood et al, 1997). Although the majority of GPs, whether they had had patients on hospital-at-home schemes ($N=55$) or not ($N=86$), believed that the schemes increased their workload, GPs who had experienced hospital-at-home were significantly more likely to say that hospital-at-home did not have any effect on their workload. In the West London schemes, GPs were meant to have the option of refusing an admission to hospital-at-home for their patients. The study found that 38% (21 out of 55) of GPs whose patients had used hospital-at-home were not aware of this option. According to these GPs, they have a substantial input into the care of patients on hospital-at-home: 49% (27 out of 55) of GPs who had had a patient on hospital-at-home had carried out a home visit, and 56% (31 out of 55) had dealt with a telephone call from their last patient on hospital-at-home. The proportions were significantly higher for prevention of admission patients compared with early discharge patients. Despite this, there was cautious support from GPs for the use of hospital-at-home, particularly for terminal care, stroke and chest infections.

The West London study underlines the difficulties that there were with the development of hospital-at-home in this area, and the resistance that the schemes met from a range of managers and professionals.

Conclusion: considerations for the development of innovations at the interface

In this chapter, innovations at the interface between primary and secondary care, particularly hospital-at-home, have been discussed. These innovations have developed out of the wider policy to shift care and resources from secondary to primary care. By analysing the experience of hospital-at-home, it is possible to draw out some general themes for the development of such innovations and for the policy to 'shift the balance' in general. This policy was an attempt at a major strategic change in the organization and management of health care. One way to analyse both the policy and the experience of hospital-at-home is to see whether the factors that promote strategic change were present. Pettigrew et al (1992), in their study of a number of different strategic changes in the NHS, such as the introduction of general management and the closure of long-stay psychiatric institutions, have identified eight interrelated factors (or 'receptive contexts') that facilitate strategic change. The West London study analysed hospital-at-home in the light of four of these factors: key people leading the change; the quality and coherence of the policy; supportive organizational culture; and co-operative interorganizational networks.

Key people achieving change

Stocking (1985), in her study of innovation diffusion in the NHS, identifies the importance of 'product champions' to explain why some innovations were adopted. Hospital-at-home schemes in West London appeared to have relatively weak product champions. They were nurse rather than doctor led, which meant that, in the context of the medically dominated NHS hierarchy, they were already at a disadvantage. Furthermore, the schemes were managed within the historically less powerful community health services providers. The relative power of the acute sector has long been recognized (Hunter, 1980).

Quality and coherence of the policy

Pettigrew et al (1992) found that a policy needs to provide quality and coherence both in analytic and process terms. In analytic terms, a policy needs to be rooted in data (i.e. evidence based); in process terms, the vision underpinning the policy needs to be shared amongst those implementing it and those who could promote or impede its implementation. The case of hospital-at-home in West London illustrates the lack of both an analytical and a process component. Because of the short lead-in time, there were no feasibility studies conducted, for example, to identify the number and types of patient who would benefit. Second, there was evidence in West London, at least initially, of confusion surrounding the objectives of hospital-at-home schemes. While senior managers in both health authorities and Trusts understood that the schemes had to fulfil the 'substitution' objective, many staff working in the schemes took longer to understand and accept this. Furthermore, the hospital-at-home schemes and the policy to shift care and resources from secondary to primary care more generally were based on an unrealistic financial framework that did not take into account the fixed costs of hospitals. Some commentators have argued that, in relation to primary care substitutes for accident and emergency services, there is, because the UK has a relatively highly developed system of primary health care, less scope to influence patient behaviour than in the USA, for example, where primary care is less well developed (Roberts and Mays, 1997). It may be that this argument can be applied to other primary care innovations that are attempting to substitute for secondary care.

Supportive organizational culture

In their study, Pettigrew et al (1992) identified features of a culture within DHAs that were associated with a high rate of change. These included flexible working across boundaries, an open, risk-taking approach, openness to research and evaluation, and a strong value base. Once again, the development of hospital-at-home in West London illustrates the lack of these. The schemes were established as separate, 'stand-alone' services that were not integrated into the main district nursing services and were perceived to have been favoured in resource terms by receiving LIZ funding. As a result, the schemes were often perceived as 'Rolls Royce' services and resented as such. Second, hospital-at-home staff and managers rarely revealed an openness to research and evaluation. On the contrary, many were fearful of the evaluation, understandably given that the future of the schemes, and therefore their jobs, was dependent on the study's findings.

Co-operative interorganizational networks

Kanter's (1985) study of change in the private sector reveals the importance of networks and their role in facilitating trust and negotiation. These networks are also important in the post-reformed NHS in which health authorities and Trusts, and different types of Trust, are separate organizations. They are particularly important at the interface between secondary and primary care as this also represents an interface between several different provider organizations (usually acute trust, community trust and general practice). The case study of hospital-at-home in West London at best revealed an absence of these co-operative networks, and at worst showed hostility between different organizations. As noted earlier, the history of poor relationships between one community health trust and its neighbouring acute hospital was a significant factor in one of the hospital-at-home scheme's low activity levels.

    This raises the issue of who should manage hospital-at-home. There is a debate about whether hospital-at-home schemes should be managed by community services ('inreach') or by acute hospitals ('outreach'), both in the UK (Husain, 1996) and the USA (Goodwin, 1992). The West London study shows that early discharge schemes run by community services trusts have to undertake a great deal of development and liaison work with hospitals, prior to setting up the scheme and for at least the first 6 months. Second, hospital-at-home uses considerable resources to recruit and identify patients, often without the assistance of ward staff, and takes responsibility for discharge arrangements traditionally arranged by the ward. This input is costly and is one of the reasons that puts hospital-at-home at a disadvantage in terms of cost compared with standard in-patient care (Hensher et al, 1996). It is important that acute hospitals are given the opportunity to manage hospital-at-home schemes to see how this compares with schemes run by community trusts.

The future

In West London, as a result of the findings of the evaluation, the funding for three early discharge schemes and one prevention of admission scheme has been discontinued. At least in this area, policy has been based on evidence. However, the growth of hospital-at-home schemes throughout the country has occurred without the evidence to support it (Shepperd and Iliffe, 1996).

While the experience of hospital-at-home in West London cannot be generalized to hospital-at-home elsewhere, there are important organizational issues that should be considered by those planning hospital-at-home or other innovations at the interface between the secondary and primary care sectors.

Health care organizations have been characterized as professionalized bureaucracies (Mintzberg, 1990) in which there can be resistance to innovation, leading to incremental decision-making (Lindblom, 1959). There are a number of studies of decision-making in health care that illustrate this incrementalism. Hunter's (1980) study of the allocation of development funds found that the pressures to maintain the policy *status quo* were more powerful than attempts to change policy, as challenges to the acute sector specialities were rarely successful, and the rhetoric of change did not result in shifts in the allocation of resources.

The West London study shows resistance to hospital-at-home from a wide range of groups, including acute clinicians and managers, GPs, acute purchasing managers, and a minority of patients. The development of hospital-at-home schemes and the 'shifting the balance' policy as a whole illustrates this tendency towards incrementalism and compartmentalization instead of whole-system thinking, that is, the consideration of health care as 'an interacting system' (Harrison, 1996). Hospital-at-home schemes and other innovations at the interface between primary and secondary care have been established on a small scale, in isolation from the system in which they operate. These innovations should be considered within the context of the continuum of care from pre-acute through acute and post-acute care. Radical reorganizations of acute care have been advocated (Harrison and Prentice, 1996), and hospital-at-home should be considered alongside other options as part of planning the hospitals of the future. Furthermore, as others have noted (Evans, 1996), the development of such innovations should take account of the political and cultural barriers to the policy of 'shifting the balance'.

References

Anand J, Pryor G (1982) Hospital at home. Health Trends 21(2): 46–8.
Audit Commission (1995) United They Stand: Co-ordinating Care for Elderly Patients with Hip Fracture. London: HMSO.

Black N (1997) Health services research: saviour or chimera? Lancet 349: 1834–6.

Boufford J (1994) Shifting the Balance from Acute to Community Health Care. London: King's Fund College.

Branger P, van't Hooft A, van der Wouden H (1995) Co-ordinating shared care using electronic data interchange. Medinfo 8(2): 1995.

Brooks R (1996) Your place or mine. Health Services Journal (25 April): 35.

Bull M (1989) GP obstetrics: making the most of shared care. Practitioner 233: 211–15.

Byers D, Parker M (1992) Early home rehabilitation for the patient with hip fracture. British Journal of Occupational Therapy 52: 351–4.

Clarke A (1996) Why are we trying to reduce the length of stay? Evaluation of the costs and benefits of reducing time in hospital must start from the objectives that govern change. Quality in Health Care 5: 172–9.

Coast J, Inglis A, Frankel S (1996) Alternatives to hospital care: what are they and who should decide? British Medical Journal 312: 162–6.

Coulter A (1995) Shifting the balance from secondary to primary care. British Medical Journal 311: 1447–8.

Currie E, Maynard A (1989) The Economics of Hospital Acquired Infection. Discussion Paper No. 56. York: University of York, Centre for Health Economics.

Dale J, Green J, Reid F, Glucksman E, Higgs R (1995) Primary care in the accident and emergency department. II: Comparison of general practitioners and hospital doctors. British Medical Journal 311: 427–30.

Department of Health (1993) Making London Better. London: HMSO.

Donald I, Neil Baldwin R, Bannerjee M (1995) Gloucester hospital at home: a randomised controlled trial. Age and Ageing 24: 434–9.

Elliot M (1995) Providing support and care through a hospital at home. Nursing Times 91(34): 36–7.

Essex B, Doig R, Renshaw J (1990) Pilot study of records of shared care for people with mental illnesses. British Medical Journal 300: 1442–6.

Evans D (1996) A stakeholder analysis of developments at the primary and secondary care interface. British Journal of General Practice 46: 675–7.

Fulop N, Hood S, Parsons S (1997) Does the National Health Service want hospital-at-home? Journal of the Royal Society of Medicine 90: 212–15.

George S, Read S, Westlake L, Fraser-Moodie A, Pritty P, Williams B (1993) Differences in priorities assigned to patients by triage nurses and by consultant physicians in accident and emergency departments. Journal of Epidemiology and Community Health 47(4): 312–15.

Goodwin S (1992) Short-term care and treatment in the home: nursing perspective. In Costain D, Warner M (Eds) From Hospital to Home. London: King's Fund.

Green J, Thorogood N (1998) Analysing Health Policy: A Sociological Approach. London: Longman.

Hallam L, Wilkin D, Roland M (1996) 24 Our Responsive Health Care. Manchester: University of Manchester, National Primary Care Research and Development Centre.

Ham C, Hunter D, Robinson R (1995) Evidence based policy making. British Medical Journal 310: 71–2.

Harris A (1994) How should changes in primary health care be evaluated? In Marinker M (Ed.) Controversies in Health Care Policies. London: BMJ Publishing Group.

Harrison A (1996) Structural change in hospitals: the implications for research. Journal of Health Services Research and Policy 1(1): 44–50.

Harrison A, Prentice S (1996) Acute Futures. London: King's Fund.

Harvey I, Jenkins R, Llewellyn L (1993) Enhancing appropriateness of acute bed use: the role of the patient hotel. Journal of Epidemiology and Community Health 47(5): 368–72.

Hensher M, Fulop N, Hood S, Ujah S (1996) Does hospital at home make economic sense? Results of an economic evaluation of early discharge hospital at home care for orthopaedic patients in three areas of West London. Journal of Royal Society of Medicine 89: 548–51.

Hollingworth W, Todd C, Parker M, Roberts J, Williams R (1993) Cost analysis of early discharge after hip fracture. British Medical Journal 307: 903–6.

Hollingworth W, Todd C, Parker M (1995) The cost of treating hip fractures in the twenty first century. Journal of Public Health Medicine 17(3): 269–76.

Hood S, Parsons S, Fulop N (1997) Evaluation of Seven Hospital at Home Schemes across North Thames Region: Final Report to North Thames R&D Organisational and Management Group London: NHS Executive North Thames Office R&D.

Hughes J, Gordon P (1993) Hospitals and Primary Care: Breaking the Boundaries 2nd Edn. London: King's Fund Centre.

Hunter D (1980). Coping with Uncertainty. Chichester: Research Studies Press.

Husain O (1996) 'Dumping' fears are starting to hit home. Doctor (15 February): 84.

Iliffe S (1997) Hospital at home: buyer beware. Journal of the Royal Society of Medicine 90(4): 181–2.

Kanter R (1985) The Change Masters: Corporate Entrepreneurs at Work. London: Allen & Unwin.

King M, Nazareth I (1996) Community care of patients with schizophrenia: the role of the primary health care team. British Journal of General Practice 46(405): 231–7.

King's Fund Centre (1989) Hospital at Home: The Coming Revolution. London: King's Fund Centre Health and Social Care Communication Unit.

King's Fund Commission on the Future of London's Acute Health Services (1992) London Health Care 2010: Changing the Future of Services in the Capital. London: King's Fund.

Knowelden J, Westlake L, Wright K, Clarke S (1991) Peterborough hospital at home: an evaluation. Journal of Public Health Medicine 13(3): 182–8.

Lindblom C (1959) The science of muddling through. Public Administration Review 38: 316–25.

Lowy A, Brazier J, Fall M, Thomas K, Jones N, Williams B (1993) Minor surgery by general practitioners under the 1990 contract: effects on hospital workload. British Medical Journal 307: 413–17.

McGhee S, McInnes G, Hedley A, Murray T, Reid J (1994) Co-ordinating and standardising long-term care: evaluation of the west of Scotland shared care scheme for hypertension. British Journal of General Practice 44(387): 441–5.

Marks L (1991) Home and Hospital Care: Redrawing the Boundaries. London: King's Fund Institute.

Mays N, Morley V, Boyle S, Newman P, Towell D (1997) Evaluating Primary Care Development: A Review of Evaluation in the London Initiative Zone Primary Care Development Programme. London: King's Fund.

Mintzberg H (1990) Mintzberg on Management. London: Free Press.

Moss F, McNicol M (1993) Secondary care beyond Tomlinson: an opportunity to be seized or squandered? In Smith J (Ed.) London after Tomlinson: Reorganising Big City Medicine. London: BMJ Publishing Group.

Mowat I, Morgan R (1982) Peterborough hospital at home scheme. British Medical Journal 284: 641–3.

National Health Service Executive (1994) Developing NHS purchasing and GP fundholding: towards a primary-care led NHS. EL(94)79. London: NHSE.

National Health Service Executive (1997) National R&D Programme in the Area of the Primary–Secondary Care Interface. Three Year Programme Report. London: NHS Executive North Thames.

O'Caithan A (1994) Evaluation of a hospital at home scheme for the discharge of patients with fractured neck of femur. Journal of Public Health Medicine 16(2): 205–10.

Parker M, Pryor G, Myles J (1991) Early discharge after hip fracture. Acta Orthopaedica Scandinavica 62(6): 563–6.

Pedersen L, Leese B (1997) What will a primary care led NHS mean for workload? The problem of the lack of an evidence base. British Medical Journal 314: 1337–41.

Petrie J, Robb O, Webster J, Scott A, Jeffers T, Park M (1985) Computer assisted shared care in hypertension. British Medical Journal of Clinical Research and Education 290: 1960–2.

Pettigrew A, Ferlie E, McKee L (1992) Shaping Strategic Change. London: Sage.

Pryor G, Williams D (1989) Rehabilitation after hip fractures. Home and hospital management combined. Journal of Bone and Joint Surgery 71(B): 471–4.

Richards S, Coast J, Gunnell D et al (1998) Randomised controlled trial comparing effectiveness and acceptability of an early discharge hospital-at-home scheme with acute hospital care. British Medical Journal 316: 1796–801.

Rink E, Sims J, Walker R, Pickard L (1998) Hospital care at home: an evaluation of a scheme for orthopaedic patients. Health and Social Care in the Community 6(3): 158–63.

Roberts E, Mays N (1997) Accident and Emergency Care at the Interface: A Systematic Review of the Evidence on Substitution. London: King's Fund.

Roberts P (1992) Hip home. Nursing Times 88(44): 28–30.

Sackett D, Rosenberg W (1995) The need for evidence-based medicine. Journal of the Royal Society of Medicine 88(11): 620–4.

Salisbury C (1997) Observational study of a general practice out of hours co-operative: measures of activity. British Medical Journal 314: 182–6.

Scott A (1996). Primary or secondary care? What can economics contribute to evaluation at the interface? Journal of Public Health Medicine 18(1): 19-26.

Secretary of State for Health (1996a) Primary care: The Future – Choice and Opportunity. London: HMSO.

Secretary of State for Health (1996b) Primary Care: Delivering the Future. London: HMSO.

Shepperd S, Iliffe S (1996) Hospital at home: an uncertain future. British Medical Journal 312: 923–4 (editorial).

Shepperd S, Iliffe S (1997) Hospital at home compared to in-patient hospital care (Review). In Bero L, Grilli R, Grimshaw J, Oxman A (Eds) Collaboration on Effective Professional Practice Module of the Cochrane Database on Systematic Reviews (updated 01 December 1997). Available in the Cochrane Library (database on disk and CDROM). The Cochrane Collaboration; Issue 1. Oxford: Update Software; 1998.

Shepperd S, Harwood D, Jenkinson C, Gray A, Vessey M, Morgan P (1998a) Randomised controlled trial comparing hospital-at-home with in-patient hospital care I: three month follow up of health outcomes. British Medical Journal 316: 1786–91.

Shepperd S, Harwood D, Gray A, Vessey M, Morgan P (1998b) Randomised controlled trial comparing hospital-at-home with in-patient hospital care II: cost minimisation analysis. British Medical Journal 316: 1791–96.

Sims J, Rink E, Walker R, Pickard L (1997) The introduction of a hospital at home service: a staff perspective. Journal of Interprofessional Care 11(2): 217–24.

Snell J (1995) Three years after Tomlinson – why millions are still unspent. Health Service Journal (12 October): 22–4.

Starfield B (1994) Is primary care essential? Lancet 344: 1129–33.

Steele R, Wootton R (1997) Primary care telemedicine in the UK. British Journal of General Practice 47(414): 4–5 (editorial).

Stocking B (1985) Innovation and inertia in the NHS London: Nuffield Provincial Hospitals Trust.

Taylor M, Readman S, Hague B, Boulter V, Hughes L, Howell S (1994) A district epilepsy service with community-based specialist liaison nurses and guidelines for shared care. Seizure 3(2): 121–7.

Tomlinson B (1992) Report of the Inquiry into Health Services, Medical Education, and Research. London: HMSO.

Van Damme R, Drummond N, Beattie J, Douglas G (1994) Integrated care for patients with asthma: views of general practitioners. British Journal of General Practice 44: 9–13.

Victor C, Nazareth B, Hudson M, Fulop N (1993) The inappropriate use of acute hospital beds in an inner London District Health Authority. Health Trends 25(3): 94–7.

Waddington E, Henwood M (1996) Going Home: An Evaluation of British Red Cross Home from Hospital Schemes. Leeds: University of Leeds, Nuffield Institute for Health.

Warner M (1996) Shifting borders: hospitals, primary health care and community care. In World Health Organisation (Ed.) European Health Care Reforms: Analysis of Current Strategies. Copenhagen: WHO.

Warner M, Riley C (1993) Closer to Home: Healthcare in the 21st Century. Birmingham: National Association of Health Authorities and Trusts.

Wilson A, Parker H, Wynn A (1997). Hospital at home is as safe as hospital, cheaper and patients like it more: early results from a randomised controlled trial. Journal of Epidemiology and Community Health Society for Social Medicine Abstacts 51(5): 593.

World Health Organisation (1996) European Health Care Reforms: Analysis of Current Strategies. Copenhagen: WHO.

Worth R, Nicholson A, Bradley P (1990) Shared care for diabetes between hospital and GPs. Nursing Times 86(41): 52.

Chapter 8
Information technology in primary care

Elizabeth Mitchell and Frank Sullivan

Introduction

The past decade has seen a major increase in the level of computerization in primary care. There are undoubted and obvious benefits to primary care workers when the powerful, dedicated and (usually) reliable memory of the computer is applied to a variety of menial and repetitive tasks, such as repeat prescribing or the maintenance of the age–sex register. The question to be addressed in this chapter is whether there is any evidence that this change has delivered any benefit to patients. To improve patient care, computers would need to be superior to the human brain in the process of decision-making. However, computers can already improve call and recall systems for preventive activities and chronic disease management when they are integrated into well-organized practices. The science of primary care informatics will develop through the careful evaluation of each new function offered by software houses by critically aware clinicians and researchers. We are likely to see clinical and strategic decision support increasing in importance as technology matures sufficiently to bring the best evidence to the point at which it is needed: the consultation (Sullivan and MacNaughton, 1996).

Origins and early uses of primary care computing

The uptake of information technology (IT) has increased at such speed over the past decade that we tend to imagine that computer use sprang up almost overnight, gathered speed in the 1980s and careered headlong into the 90s. In fact, the development and evaluation of primary care computing has been going on for over 30 years.

Some of the earliest work was carried out in Oxford, as part of the Oxford Record Linkage Study, which was set up to demonstrate whether or not it was practical, or indeed beneficial, to collate patient health data. The information that had previously been held by a variety of health professionals could now be contained in one centralized record (Acheson, 1964). Data were batch-processed on a remote mainframe computer. In 1968, one general practice was used to study how this information could be retrieved (Acheson and Forbes, 1968). The experiment was later rolled out to several other practices who collectively took part in the Oxford Community Health Project (Perry, 1972).

The idea of an information system for a complete health centre was first reported by Abrams et al in 1968. The purpose of their study was to provide doctors and other health professionals with a user-friendly system that would allow them to insert information during consultations and obtain rapid access to the record. Eventually, a fully operational system was set up at a health centre in Thamesmead (Abrams, 1972). In 1969, a project was established in Livingston New Town that set out to establish a computer-assisted medical records system and to monitor the effects of this on personnel. The system recorded registration data and episode data, which the doctor taped on a dictaphone after each patient contact. This information was then transcribed by a coding clerk before it was entered into the computer (Gruer and Heasman, 1970). Collecting episode data did not involve much work for the doctors and in fact made them more disciplined in systematic recording. However, coding this information proved very time-consuming and took up around one-quarter of secretarial time.

These early computer studies had all depended on the remote batch-processing of data. In 1970, the first experiment using a real-time data system was conducted (Preece et al, 1970; Lippman and Preece, 1971). This IBM desktop pilot scheme established the use of visual display units (VDUs), through which the doctor and his secretary had immediate access to a computer 180 miles away for 3 hours each night via a post office telecommunications line. Many of the aspects of computerized medical records that we recognize today, such as patient history, repeat medication and recall for immunization, originated from this system.

The Exeter Project (Bradshaw-Smith, 1976) also used a real-time data system but attempted to take the idea one step further. The aim of the project was to make patient records accessible not only to the GP, but also to other health professionals such as hospital consultants, nursing staff and even service departments. Participating practices were linked by telecommunication lines to a mainframe computer based at the Computer Centre of the Royal Exeter and Devon Hospitals. Use of the system began in 1976 and was met with mixed reviews from participants. Some found the computerized record advantageous: it could be updated immediately, saved time and was more flexible than paper records (Bradshaw-Smith, 1976). Others felt that the disadvantages of the new system – learning new skills, time, cost, system breakdowns and intrusion on the doctor–patient relationship – outweighed its advantages (Bolden, 1981). Although justified at the time, the improvement of technology and experience was to overcome most if not all of these problems.

Most of the early research dealt with the use of computers for the collection and administration of routine patient data, but work was also being carried out on the use of computers for activities more directly related to patient care, such as disease prevention. One GP had already established a register of all 16 000 patients in his practice, which was used to invite people to screening and immunization programmes such as those for diabetes and cervical cytology, and middle-age clinics (Hodes, 1968). Also around this time, an Edinburgh GP began using a computer to record morbidity data, which involved recording up to four diagnoses for each consultation. At the end of each month, the GP transferred the original paper record on to punched paper tape, which was transferred on to magnetic tape at the end of 1 year (Dinwoodie, 1969). By the early 1970s, practitioners began to use their computers not only to record practice activity, but also to audit it (Johnson, 1972; Durno, 1973).

Growth of computing in the UK

Although computers had been around primary care since the 1960s, it was not until the 1980s, and the latter part of the decade in particular, that their uptake became widespread. The RCGP has been in favour of computers since its Computer Working Party, which was established in 1978, published a report considering 'the desirability and practicability of the use of computers for general practice clinical records' and reporting on 'recommendations for future development' (Royal College of General Practitioners, 1980).

However, the government's 'Micros for GPs' scheme, launched in 1982, was the first real step towards universal general practice computerization. This scheme was initiated by the Department of Trade and Industry as part of Information Technology Year, IT-82. Under the scheme, 150 practices in Britain received 50% of the cost of installing a particular computer system (either CAP (UK) or British Medical Data Systems). The systems allowed patient registration, repeat prescribing and screening and recall. In return for this technology, practices agreed to participate in an evaluation of its use over a 3-year period. Although the scheme attracted criticism at the time, mainly over the lack of choice of available computer systems, 2000 practices were interested in participating. This scheme was probably the first to alert both GPs themselves and the commercial companies to the possibility of a real market for GP computing systems.

In 1987, VAMP and AAH Meditel, two of the largest computer suppliers in the country, introduced no-cost schemes whereby practices were offered free multi-user computer systems. These practices would then provide the companies with anonymous patient data on morbidity and repeat prescribing. In this way, large databases of regularly updated health information would be created and these could, in turn, be sold to the pharmaceutical industry as a way of recouping the cost of the free systems. As a result of this partnership, 19% of practices were computerized by 1988 and 28% by 1989 (Department of Health, 1993).

In Scotland, the situation was somewhat different. After the 'Micros for GPs' scheme ended, the 17 Scottish practices that had taken part were concerned that the progress and enthusiasm that had been created towards computerization in Scotland would fall away just as the interest of the companies providing the systems had done. To prevent this, David Ferguson, a Glasgow GP, offered them a software package that he had originally designed for repeat prescribing. The subsequent development of the General Practice Administration System Scotland (GPASS) has been financially supported by the Scottish Home and Health Department. GPASS has been offered free to any practice with compatible hardware since 1984. Encouraged by this incentive, the number of computerized practices in Scotland rose to 27% by 1988 and 36% by 1989, covering more than one-third of the population of Scotland (Ryan, 1989).

Also during the 1980s came the development of the READ code classification, the first system of morbidity codes designed to standardize medical information on computer (General Medical Services Committee/Royal College of General Practitioners, 1988). The codes are structured in a five-level (originally four-level) alphanumeric hierarchy, in which each character is linked to the specific category for which it is an alternative term. The first character denotes the grouping [C... Endoc/nutr/metab/immune diseases], and the remaining characters branch out within that grouping until the required detail is reached [C1... Other endocrine gland disorder; C10... Diabetes mellitus; C105... Diabetes + eye manifestation; C1051... Diabetes + eye manifest – adult]. The READ classification codes over 25 000 medical conditions and procedures, extensively covering diagnoses, procedures and medications as well as demographics, history and symptoms and diagnostic tests. The DoH purchased the READ classification in 1990 and established a National Coding Centre to maintain and develop the system.

Undoubtedly the most compelling spur in the drive towards computerization came in the shape of the 1990 contract for NHS GPs. Greater emphasis was now placed on health promotion, identification of at risk groups and disease prevention. In an attempt to ensure that these obligations were met by practitioners, remuneration was linked to the targets met. These included targets for the proportion of children vaccinated, the proportion of cervical smears carried out, child health surveillance, health promotion clinics and annual checkups for the over-75s. Practices now had to send annual reports to their health authorities detailing all of these activities, and regular audit was to be undertaken by all practices. In order to receive maximum payment for their activity, practices had to identify all those requiring immunization, smears, over-75 assessments and so on. Not only did they need to identify groups of patients by age and sex, but they now also had to identify them by condition. They needed to know who required screening and when they needed it, and they had to regularly monitor their own performance. The introduction of fundholding also enabled selected practices to control their own budgets, making them responsible for purchasing any services that they required for their patients, paying their own personnel and prescribing costs. Practices that became fundholders also had to keep up to date with the finances of the practice and the purchasing of hospital services.

It would be difficult to produce all of this information without the aid of some type of automated information system. As part of the contract, the DoH offered a 50% reimbursement on the acquisition and running costs of computer systems. This may explain the rapid increase in the number of computerized practices from 1990 onwards (Figure 8.1). In 1989, only 28% of practices had a computer. This increased to 47% with the introduction of the contract and to 63% in the following year. The NHSME survey (Department of Health, 1993) predicted that by 1997, over 90% of practices would be computerized.

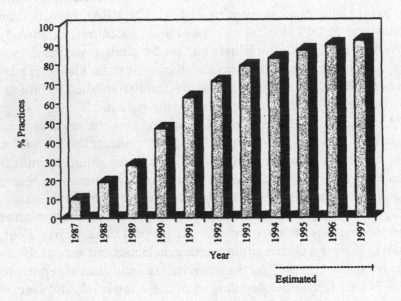

Figure 8.1: Percentage of practices using computers in the UK
Source: NHS Management Executive Computerisation in GP Practices, 1993 survey (Department of Health, 1993).

The increase in the popularity of computing systems also created an increase in costs. The average cost of purchasing a computer system rose from around £10 000 in 1990/91 to almost £15 000 in 1993, with annual maintenance costs averaging between £1300 and £2400 over the same period (Department of Health, 1993). At 1997 prices, purchasing a system would therefore cost between £12 100 and £18 200, and maintaining it between £1580 and £2900. Reimbursing practices for this outlay for the first 4 years since the introduction of the NHS Information Management and Technology strategy for primary care in 1990 has cost the government almost £1.5 billion (NHS Management Executive, personal communications, 1994).

Uses and users of primary care IT

So, computers have been in existence in primary care for over 30 years and have been present in most general practices for almost a decade. The concept of the linked patient record has been mastered, and advances in hardware and software have provided members of the primary health care team with technology allowing rapid access to the complete history of any patient in their practice. Computers now have the ability to collate and sort patient data and 'flag' patient files to highlight particular issues or act as a reminder to perform a particular task. They allow practices to set up their own drug formularies, use protocols of care, and interact with hospital departments and pathology laboratories using e-mail links. They have the capacity to provide not only referral letters and referral recording, but also referral appointment-making. There is even the ability to access remote databases that provide reference materials, ranging from Medline searching to guidelines.

More than half of the GPs in Britain have a desktop computer on their desk, but aside from the 'computer buffs', computer use is still generally administrative, with patient registration, repeat prescribing and screening, and recall the three main functions carried out (Richards and Sullivan, 1996). In its most recent survey, the DoH found that almost all computerized practices used the computer for patient registration and repeat prescribing (98% and 94% respectively). Using the computer for call and recall was commonplace (84% of practices), as was carrying out audit tasks (77% of practices). Many practices used the computer to flag records (63%), issue acute prescriptions (58%) and produce referral letters (51%) (Department of Health, 1993) (Figure 8.2). In Scotland, figures were somewhat similar (Taylor et al, 1992), although it appears that more use is made of the clinical record-keeping capabilities of the computer (46%), whilst flagging records (25%) and producing referral letters (22%) are not as popular. In the UK as a whole, referring to electronic protocols of care or using the computer for research purposes does not yet seem to be a very common occurrence.

The use of computers as primarily information management tools is perhaps a reflection of the main groups of primary care staff who use computers within practices (Table 8.1). Receptionists and secretaries are two of the largest user groups, which surely explains the high proportion of practices using the computer for patient registration data and, indeed, the call and recall facilities, since these groups will undoubtedly identify patients and invite them for screening.

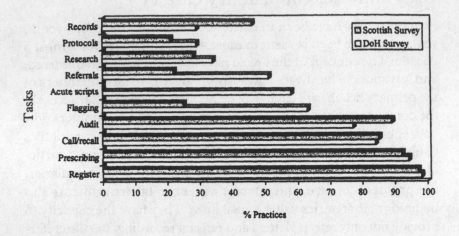

Figure 8.2: Tasks carried out with computers in primary care in the UK
Sources: NHS Management Executive Computerisation in GP Practices, 1993 survey (Department of Health), 1993; Taylor et al (1992).

Table 8.1: Computer users within practices in the UK

User	% Practices	
	Department of Health survey (1993)	Taylor et al survey (1992)
Doctors	80	70
Practice nurses	76	45
Receptionists	92	91
Secretaries	65	59
Practice managers	82	62
Fundholding staff	5	2
Attached nurses	8	7
Attached health visitors	11	13

Sources: NHS Management Executive Computerisation in GP Practices, 1993 survey (Department of Health, 1993); Taylor et al (1992).

Doctors, as another main user group, are responsible for the high level of repeat prescribing carried out. However, what is surprising is that, except for practice nurses in England and Wales, very few of the nursing groups within practices appear to use the computer. This group would unquestionably provide a wealth of relevant and useful patient data, not only clinical, but also social. Perhaps their lack of computer utilization is a statement about the design of the systems that have a primarily administrative-based rather than patient-based focus. Articles such as the those in the 1995 *British Medical Journal* series 'ABC of medical computing' (Millman et al, 1995a, 1995b, 1995c) and in the nursing press (Mongiardi and Dirckze, 1995; Hammond et al, 1997), which describe the functions available to the primary health care team, may go some way to reducing this imbalance amongst user groups.

The impact of IT on primary care

Users have been trying to evaluate the effects of IT since it was first introduced into primary care. Investigators are still involved in the same process. Perhaps the very nature of this technology means that we will constantly be striving to keep up. No sooner have we evaluated one system or aspect of a system than everything has changed: technology has moved on and the system needs to be re-evaluated. The rapid increase in the proportion of computerized practices over the past few years has not helped this dilemma. The very fact that so many practices are computerized should urge us to ensure that systems are utilized in the best possible way, so that they can provide some benefit for patients. On the other hand, as there are now so few practices in Britain without computers, evaluating their use often seems futile since practices are unlikely to abandon their computers and go back to a completely paper-based system. Thus, the way forward must be the continual evaluation of the one area of primary care where computers can have the most impact, both positive and negative – the consultation. Research on this particular aspect of computerization covers three broad areas:

1. the consultation itself: its duration, its structure and the doctor–patient relationship;
2. the practitioners: what they do and how often;
3. the patients: their health status and satisfaction.

Computers in the consultation

As long ago as 1969, practitioners were voicing their concerns over the impact that computers might have on the consultation (Marinker, 1969). Marinker was concerned that computers would lead doctors to 'sum up a consultation with the title of a disease', thus reducing the consultation to merely an interaction between a doctor and a condition rather than the literally unique occasion between a patient, the doctor and the illness. This early anxiety over a loss to the doctor–patient relationship may not have been completely unfounded.

In one Nottinghamshire practice, methods were developed that would allow classification of the verbal interaction and other activities that took place during consultations whilst computers were in use (Pringle et al, 1985, 1986). The analysis of a number of video-recorded consultations showed that computers seemed to lead to a more doctor-centred rather than patient-centred consultation. Medical topics raised by the doctor and tasks carried out increased, as did the proportion of the consultation that was taken up with the doctor speaking. This resulted in a reduction in patient-initiated topics and speech. It is also possible for doctors to become so involved with using the computer that they can 'forget' to communicate with the patient (Herzmark et al, 1984); hopefully, this is more because of a lack of familiarity with the technology rather than the desire to communicate with the computer and not the patient.

One benefit of a hand-written patient record is the time taken to document the result of a consultation. Doctors will scribble a few lines during or after the consultation, lasting no more than a few minutes, sometimes only seconds. Using a computer usually means extra administration – recording information in the electronic patient record while still recording it in the paper record. This has a knock-on effect on the length of the consultation, which has been seen to increase by as much as 1.5 minutes (Weingarten et al, 1989). This increase in consultation length may be to an individual patient's benefit if the doctor is being prompted to carry out preventive activities, but ultimately 'each minute added to the average consultation means over 100 extra hours a year for the average doctor. This must either be an addition to his normal workload or must squeeze the patient's consulting time' (Pringle, 1987).

Clinicians' response to computers

Primary care deals with a wide variety of different concerns, on both a clinical and a social level. The presenting complaint is often not the problem that led the patient to consult with his doctor in the first place. As a result, the consultation can be complex and may, as such, not always lend itself to complete computerization. However, computers do have the ability to bring order to the highly structured aspects of the consultation, and it is here that they can provide valuable support for the clinician. One of the most frequently used facilities of primary care computing is repeat prescribing. This function means that receptionists will spend less time processing prescriptions, and doctors will spend less time issuing and completing them (Roland et al, 1985). This not only provides patients and pharmacists with a legible prescription, but also allows the practice to monitor prescribing patterns, with the aim of increasing generic prescribing and subsequently reducing costs (Donald, 1986, 1989).

Doctors and nurses working in primary care usually define their role as that of a 'problem-solver', reacting to the problems that their patients present to them. Pringle's work, which demonstrated that computers can direct doctors to more 'medical' content, has been confirmed by further research. A wide variety of screening and preventive work may be increased by computer prompting (Sullivan and Mitchell, 1995). Using a computer to print a reminder message to the physician at the time of consultation, or to generate a list of suitable patients for the nurse to contact, has been shown to significantly increase the uptake rate of blood pressure screening and cervical screening. McDowell et al (1989a, 1989b) found that blood pressure screening increased by 3.0–9.6%, whilst cervical screening increased by 2.4–6.3%. Other systems have developed the computerized medical record to play an active role in patient care, for example the computer reminding doctors about any patient conditions that need attention (McDonald et al, 1984). Here, the computer's ability to 'decide' was controlled by 1491 physician-authored rules that could generate 751 different reminders on subjects including 15 preventive care actions, tests required to identify existing problems, the treatment of existing problems or prophylactic treatments. Physicians using the system carried out 14–20% more study actions than did physicians in the control group, who did not receive any reminders (McDonald et al, 1984). The idea of issuing prompts can also be extended to the patient and can take the form of patient-only reminders or physician and patient reminders. The uptake of preventive services is often increased, more so when both the patient and the doctor receive a reminder (Ornstein et al, 1991).

Patient outcomes

Perhaps the most contentious issue surrounding computerization in any field of medicine is whether or not it provides any real benefits for patients in terms of outcomes of care, yet this is an area in which, over the years, little hard evidence has been produced. We now know that there is no reduction in patient satisfaction when the doctor uses a computer (Sullivan et al, 1992).

Although overall satisfaction is unaffected, there can be variations resulting from the different ways in which clinicians use the computer. It can be integrated into the consultation in such a way that the patient is directly involved (Ridsdale and Hudd, 1994) or it can be used in such a discrete way that the patient may not even be aware that it is being used at all (Solomon and Dechter, 1995). Computers have been used to help manage a variety of conditions in primary care, but showing an association between process measures of care and improved patient outcomes has proved difficult. Using computers to support the management of hypertension can lead to a reduction not only in the diastolic blood pressure of moderate hypertensives, but also in the number of consultations (McAlister et al, 1986). However, considerable doubt remains over the exact benefits and negative effects of computers on patient health outcomes. This is an area in which future research will be of great value.

Confidentiality of data

The most frequently heard criticism regarding primary care computing is over the issue of patient confidentiality; indeed, this has been the case since computers were first used (Dinwoodie, 1970). Although patients do not appear to have any problem accepting the computer as a part of the consultation, they are nevertheless worried that it is easier for people outside the surgery to gain access to their files (Rethans et al, 1988). This is especially true regarding personal information, which many patients would be reluctant to speak frankly about if it were being recorded on computer (Potter, 1981).

As part of a larger study looking at the impact of desktop computers in six Scottish practices, we recently interviewed 42 patients to get an idea of how they felt about the use of computers in primary care. The majority of patients in both the computerized and control groups said that they would not mind if their doctor used a computer during consultations. They felt that it would not interfere with the doctor–patient relationship, and despite the fact that it would not influence what they told the doctor, the main concern of patients in both groups was confidentiality, although fewer people were worried by this after 1 year (Mitchell et al, 1996). This attitude may have been influenced by the fact that, of the 17 patients who had seen their doctor use the computer, only one of them had been told what it was being used for. Surely then, we cannot be surprised if people are still concerned over the use of this technology. If it is to be accepted as useful not only to clinicians, but also to patients, we must first alleviate unfounded fears by explaining its function and connection to any external computers.

Educational packages

Health professionals working in primary care often need more information than they or their immediate working environment can provide. This is an inevitable consequence of an ever-expanding knowledge base and the human incapacity to remember everything about anything. In one study of doctors, two pieces of information that they did not currently possess were needed for every three patients whom they had seen; unfortunately, most of their needs remained unmet (Covell et al, 1985). This is partly because paper-based sources remain difficult to access and the type of electronic information available is complex. With effort, however, it is possible to discover 'patient-oriented evidence that matters' – POEMs (Slawson and Shaughnessy, 1997). These take specific problems that are of concern to the patient, find the best evidence (with patient-oriented outcomes) and present it in a digestible format to practising clinicians. The importance of this subject also relates to the fact that traditional approaches to continuing education are relatively ineffective (Sibley et al, 1982). Many doctors read available medical literature for up to 4 hours per week (Pickup et al, 1983), but even the most dedicated primary care practitioner cannot critically appraise and assimilate the deluge of evidence presented on a daily or a weekly basis. Recent approaches to education in primary care (to be discussed further in Chapter 10) emphasize a more problem-based approach in which computers can be of great assistance (Pendleton, 1995). The focus of this section will be on four of the most commonly used methods: computer-assisted learning (CAL), telemedicine, access to sources of evidence-based medicine and decision support systems.

Computer-assisted learning

CAL describes any system whereby information of potential educational value is provided electronically (Kidd et al, 1992). The most common forms rely upon CD-ROM, but older versions may be based on floppy disks. The most recent are accessed via the Internet. One example is the CTI Centre for Medicine (http://www.cticm.bristol.ac.uk/). This Centre, based at the University of Bristol, was established to encourage and support the use of computers in medical education. Systems may vary greatly in complexity. Advances in data communication technologies mean that multi-media information can be transported rapidly to various clinical care locations.

Many systems enable users to move from the topic of immediate concern that has been checked through highlighted terms known as 'hypertext'. This is the ability to move from one page to another by selecting the highlighted words. For example, if the package were dealing with the side-effects of oral hypoglycaemic drugs, there might be a link to other causes of hypoglycaemia; if the package were considering the optimization of inhaler techniques, there might be a link to the evidence for the value of self-monitoring. In either case, the user may be able to obtain information on the use of more recent therapeutic agents.

Some versions of CAL are designed to be appropriate for patients. Interactive programs are able to provide diagnostic or therapeutic suggestions to patients with minor ailments or more severe conditions (e.g. men contemplating prostate surgery) or chronic diseases such as diabetes and asthma.

Telemedicine

The essential feature of telemedicine is the exchange of information between two geographically separate locations, be that information voice, image or part of a medical record. Of course, doctors and nurses conducted remote consultations long before the term 'telemedicine' had been coined, usually by diagnosing and advising sick patients over the telephone. The follow-up of patients is also often possible by telephone. Voice mail systems permit telephone users to record, store or send spoken messages. These messages can be sent when it is more convenient to use a recording than to speak directly. Telemedicine can be useful in assisting hospital-at-home schemes (see Chapter 7).

A recent feature of telemedicine is the technological advance that creates a fast, two-way electronic network for interactive communication. This version of telemedicine was initially conceived as a method of providing communication links between medical experts (e.g. dermatologists or trauma surgeons) and less expert clinicians in remote locations (e.g. GPs on remote Scottish islands or paramedics on oil rigs). However, its role is now being considered as a method of reducing costs. Once again, comparisons of costs as well as benefits will be needed before the exact place of this technology in primary care is established (Maclean et al, 1997).

Access to sources of evidence-based practice

The process of evidence-based practice may be considered in four phases. The problem to be studied should be clearly identified and the evidence found and then appraised before being put into practice and having its outcomes monitored (Sackett et al, 1997). Many computer systems now include a variety of on-line resources that assist this process. These usually allow individual primary care workers to call up specific information about a particular problem, disease or drug.

For example, one may want to know whether offering elderly persons living in the community an annual comprehensive geriatric assessment reduces admission to long-term nursing home care. A review in the journal *Evidence-Based Medicine* (1996) showed that, over a 3-year period, the rate of hospital admission without the assessment service was 10% but only 4% if the service were present. This may be analysed by saying that the relative risk reduction (RRR) was 58%, or perhaps more usefully that the absolute risk reduction (ARR) was 6%. Even more beneficial is appraisal of the evidence to say that the number needed to treat (NNT, i.e. the reciprocal of ARR, 1/0.06) to prevent one long-term admission is 17. Interactive packages to enable these calculations, such as 'Catmaker' from the NHS Research and Development Centre for Evidence Based Medicine, are already available. The technology to help with these calculations is therefore available. The techniques for practising in a more evidence-based fashion (Sackett et al, 1997) are within the grasp of most primary care professionals but are best learned in a practical setting such as an evidence-based journal club or course.

Decision support

At present, the human brain is the best method of decision-making for the myriad complexity of problems that patients present to us. However, that brain is less efficient than the computer for some tasks we face; for example, it never forgets to file a smear report or issue a drug interaction warning. As a result, computers will be increasingly relied upon to provide decision support.

Strategic decision support is based outside the consultation, where professionals can use computers to review the health needs, patterns of care and outcomes for patients. Query programs such as MiQuest (Neal et al, 1996) interrogate the practice database, and adding other knowledge can unlock the potential information within these data. Incorporating risk factor scores (Jackson et al, 1993) or applications of underlying theory, for example the 'rule of halves' in hypertension detection and management (Tudor Hart, 1992), enables the identification and targeting of specific groups and individuals on whom the practice might concentrate during the next quarter. Data may be aggregated from several practices and added to other public data sources from social work, hospitals, local government and economic data on prescribing (Morris et al, 1997). This results in more streamlined services to patients, for example those with chronic obstructive airways disease, diabetes and renal failure who should have influenza and pneumococcal vaccination in the autumn, or known hypertensives who are poorly controlled at any time.

Clinical decision support aids decisions about individual patients at the time of consultation. The aim of decision support systems is to provide a set of tools that allows a clinician to access up-to-date guidelines and then apply them to the management of patients. Simple protocol systems are already appearing (Purves, 1996). Most clinical decision support systems currently focus on a relatively narrow range of diagnostic or therapeutic problems (Wyatt and Walton, 1996). Such systems may be passive, giving information only when sought; an example is the electronic *British National Formulary* or guidelines that are accessible but remain in the background until called up by the user. More active systems offer preferred prescribing suggestions with varying levels of justification, or prevent referral unless all mandatory fields in a referral decision support are completed.

Even when guidelines are available, health professionals forget to follow them. This should not be surprising as humans have a finite capacity to process complex information (Sullivan and MacNaughton, 1996) and the immaturity of current technology means that it is often difficult to access decision support quickly enough for it to be useful (Covell et al, 1985). As IT advances, and with more powerful information retrieval systems integrated into clinical computer systems, we anticipate a situation in which decision support becomes an accepted and then an expected feature of good clinical care.

The Future

This may be considered along three dimensions:

- possibility: driven by research into the sciences of informatics and telematics;
- capability: the development of scientific ideas into technological reality;
- desirability: that which will improve patient care.

The first dimension is determined by forces outside the control of the primary health care team. The second is partly determined by hardware and software manufacturers and partly by users. By specifying what we need from IT, we may be able to influence what is designed, produced and implemented. Aspects of that future that are relevant to the primary health care team are our interface with patients, primary–secondary care links and universal medical records.

Interface with patients

One example of new technology at the patient interface is the 'smart card' (see Chapter 6). Smart cards are currently being used and evaluated in a number of sites (Lavoie et al, 1995). Their use is greatest in countries where the insurance component of health care is more prominent. Smart cards are the same size as credit cards and function like the other smart cards we have become used to, for example supermarket loyalty cards. They may be used to store and transfer data between a variety of primary (and secondary) care sites with either the patient or health professional using them. Patients are now just as likely to have access to the Internet as are members of the primary health care team. Some may be sophisticated users of a variety of information sources. As more patients obtain access to electronic mail, this will offer further avenues for innovative health services.

Primary–secondary care links

The rapid communication of laboratory imaging and hospital discharge information using existing electronic data transfer mechanisms is potentially beneficial. The communication process is achieved via a modem (*modulator-demo*dulator) using the telephone lines between sites. A crucial aspect of any record linkage is security, and data encryption and password protection need to be assured.

It is likely that pilot work, such as 'Links' in England and Wales and 'Partners' in Scotland, will become part of the NHS computer network. The NHS computer network received high profile and endorsement in the government's recent White Paper *The New NHS* (Secretary of State for Health, 1997). These systems will provide the possibility of a shared health service record, allowing primary care team members access to information that is currently unattainable or difficult to obtain. The NHS Information Management and Technology strategy, which states that 'information should be person based; systems should be integrated; management information should be derived from operational clinical systems; data should be secure and confidential; and data should be shared across the NHS' (Leaning, 1993), can only be enhanced by such links.

Universal medical records

Universal medical records are those shared by all health care professionals dealing with an individual client or patient. Some would expand that definition to include other professionals working with individuals, such as social workers or voluntary agencies. There are many practice settings where doctors and nurses share the same electronic (and paper) records, but apart from amongst these two groups and administrative support staff, there is not usually any access to those records. Similarly, team members who are not employed by practices rarely share their records with the doctors and nurses. There are formidable barriers to the development of such records as long as the culture remains multi-disciplinary, with a variety of professionals working together but within separate areas. If we become interdisciplinary, with much more patient care being shared, the value of a single record system then becomes increasingly apparent.

In order for universal record systems to operate effectively, there must be agreement in three main areas. First, we need a consensus on the basic data that should be included for identification, demographics, problem definition and intervention coding. READ codes offer a means of using the same language within the NHS. Second, we need to control access to the records with passwords permitting access to those who need to know certain data items. Finally, we need adequate protection to ensure that data are secure within teams and between teams and the outside world. Encryption systems exist to allow this.

Making primary care practitioners reliant on expensive informatics systems may reduce the range of specialists to whom they can refer, which may in turn lead to technology 'lock in': a dependence on technological support may encourage other clinical skills to atrophy. We also need to measure the ancillary resources required to install and maintain the equipment and train primary care professionals in its use, to ensure that resources are not merely made available to enthusiasts.

Searching on the Internet

Guidance on searching the Internet and details of some useful websites for primary care users are given in the Appendix. The importance of utilizing websites as a means of obtaining and reviewing useful information is receiving widespread recognition. Advice, not only on the best ways to use the sites once they have been accessed (Greenhalgh, 1997), but also on their use as a means of managing clinical data (Fraser et al, 1997), is now readily available. The Internet also may prove a useful resource to the health professionals who are to run the national patient helpline proposed in the White Paper *The New NHS* (Secretary of State for Health, 1997).

Conclusion

Primary care is an information-hungry environment, and there can be no doubt that advancing IT capability will be able to satisfy some of that need. The challenge facing individuals and teams working in the community is to recognize when and how to take appropriate action. The recent legislation in Scotland (Scottish Office, 1997), England and Wales (Secretary of State for Health, 1997) has increased the demands on health service informatics. The aspiration to high-quality, effective care that is patient centred can only be delivered by a system that incorporates high-quality, primary care computing. This chapter has provided an historical framework and a description of current functionality. Hopefully, the consideration of the issues raised in these sections will allow readers to decide which of the developing ideas should enter their workplace. Telemedicine, evidence-based resources and decision support may appear desirable or inevitable, but they may also appear threatening or impossible. Understanding the scientific principles upon which they are based is likely to make them more acceptable and valuable to health workers and patients.

References

Abrams M E (1972) Health services and the computer – real time computing in general practice. Health Trends 4: 18.

Abrams M E, Bowden K F, Chamberlain J (1968) A computer-based general practice and health centre information system. Journal of the Royal College of General Practitioners 16: 415–27.

Acheson E D (1964) The Oxford record linkage study: a central file of morbidity and mortality. Records for a pilot population. British Journal of Preventive and Social Medicine 18: 8–13.

Acheson E D, Forbes J A (1968) Experiment in the retrieval of information in general practice. A preliminary report. British Journal of Preventive and Social Medicine 22: 105.

Bolden K J (1981) Computers in the consulting room. Update 23: 1627–33.

Bradshaw-Smith J H (1976) A computer record keeping system in general practice. British Medical Journal 1: 1395–7.

Covell D G, Uman G C, Manning P R (1985) Information needs in office practice: are they being met? Annals of Internal Medicine 103: 596–9.

Department of Health (1993) Computerisation in GP Practices, 1993 Survey. Leeds: NHSME.

Dinwoodie H P (1969) An elementary use of a computer for morbidity recording in general practice. Health Bulletin 27: 6–14.

Dinwoodie H P (1970) Simple computer facilities in general practice. A study of the problems involved. Journal of the Royal College of General Practitioners 19: 269–81.

Donald J B (1986) On line prescribing by computer. British Medical Journal 292: 937–9.

Donald J B (1989) Prescribing costs when computers are used to issue all prescriptions. British Medical Journal 299: 28–30.

Durno D (1973) A method of data collection in general practice. Update 7: 1153–60.

Evidence-Based Medicine (1996) 1(3): 87. Abstract of: Stuck A E, Aronow H U, Steiner A et al (1995) A trial of annual in-home comprehensive geriatric assessments for elderly people living in the community. New England Journal of Medicine 233: 1184–9.

Fraser H S F, Kohane I S, Long W J (1997) Using the technology of the world wide web to manage clinical information. British Medical Journal 314: 1600–4.

General Medical Services Committee/Royal College of General Practitioners Joint Computing Group (1988) The Classification of General Practice Data: Final Report of the GMSC/RCGP. Joint Computing Group Technical Working Party. London: GMSC, BMA.

Greenhalgh T (1997) How to read a paper. The Medline database. British Medical Journal 315: 180–3.

Gruer K T, Heasman M A (1970) Livingston New Town – use of a computer in general practice medical recording. British Medical Journal 2: 89–91.

Hammond W E, Hales J W, Lobach D F, Straube M J (1997) Integration of a computer-based patient record system into the primary care setting. Computers in Nursing 15(2): S61–8.

Herzmark G, Brownbridge G, Fitter M, Evans A (1984) Consultation use of a computer by general practitioners. Journal of the Royal College of General Practitioners 34: 649–54.

Hodes C (1968) Screening in general practice. Lancet 1: 1304–6.

Jackson R, Barham P, Bills J et al (1993) Management of raised blood pressure in New Zealand: a discussion document. British Medical Journal 307: 107–10.

Johnson R A (1972) Computer analysis of the complete medical record. Journal of the Royal College of General Practitioners 22: 655–60.

Kidd M R, Cesnik B, Connoley G, Carson N E (1992) Computer-assisted learning in medical education. Medical Journal of Australia 156: 780–2.

Lavoie G, Tremblay L, Durant P, Papillon M J, Berube J, Fortin J P (1995) Medicarte software developed for the Quebec microprocessor health card project. Medinfo 8(2): 1662.

Leaning M S (1993) The new information technology and management strategy of the NHS. British Medical Journal 307: 217.

Lippman E O, Preece J F (1971) A pilot on-line data system for general practitioners. Computers in Biomedical Research 4: 390–406.

McAlister N H, Covey H D, Tong C, Lee A, Wigle E D (1986) Randomised controlled trial of computer assisted management of hypertension in primary care. British Medical Journal 293: 670–4.

McDonald C J, Hui S L, Smith D M et al (1984) Reminders to physicians from an introspective medical record. A two-year randomised trial. Annals of Internal Medicine 100: 130–8.

McDowell I, Newell C, Rosser W (1989a) Computerised reminders to encourage cervical screening in family practice. Journal of Family Practice 28(4): 420–4.

McDowell I, Newell C, Rosser W (1989b) A randomised trial of computerised reminders for blood pressure screening in primary care. Medical Care 27: 297–305.

Maclean J R, Ritchie L D, Grant A M (1997) Telemedicine: 'communication' by any other name? British Journal of General Practice 47: 200–1.

Marinker M L (1969) Computers in general practice. Practitioner 203: 285–93.

Millman A, Lee N, Brooke A (1995a) ABC of medical computing: computers in general practice – I. British Medical Journal 311: 800–2.

Millman A, Lee N, Brooke A (1995b) ABC of medical computing: computers in general practice – II. British Medical Journal 311: 864–7.

Millman A, Lee N, Brooke A (1995c) ABC of medical computing: computers in general practice – III. British Medical Journal 311: 938–41.

Mitchell E, Sullivan F M, Murray T S, Howie J G R (1996) The Impact of Information Technology on General Practitioner Consultations in Scotland. Report for the Clinical Resource and Audit Group of the Scottish Office Home and Health Department by the Department of General Practice, University of Glasgow.

Mongiardi F, Dirckze S (1995) Making sense of IT... practice nurses and computers. Practice Nurse 10(6): 398, 400–1.

Morris A D, Boyle D I R, MacAlpine R (1997) The diabetes audit and research in Tayside Scotland (DARTS) study: electronic record linkage to create a diabetes register. British Medical Journal 315: 524–8.

Neal R D, Heywood P L, Morley S (1996) Real world data-retrieval and validation of consultation data from four general practices. Family Practice 13(5): 455–61.

Ornstein S M, Garr D R, Jenkins R G, Rust P F, Arnon A (1991) Computer-generated patient reminders. Tools to improve population adherence to selected preventive services. Journal of Family Practice 32: 82–90.

Pendleton D (1995) Professional development in general practice: problems puzzles and paradigms. British Journal of General Practice 45: 377–81.

Perry J (1972) Medical information systems in general practice. A community health project. Proceedings of the Royal Society of Medicine 65: 241.

Pickup A J, Mee L J, Hedley A J (1983) The general practitioner in continuing education. Journal of the Royal College of General Practitioners 33: 486–90.

Potter A R (1981) Computers in general practice: the patient's voice. Journal of the Royal College of General Practitioners 31: 683–5.

Preece J F, Gillings D B, Lippman E O, Pearson N G (1970) An on-line medical record maintenance and retrieval system in general practice. International Journal of Biomedical Computing 1: 329–37.

Pringle M (1987) Greeks bearing gifts. British Medical Journal 295: 738–9.

Pringle M, Robins S, Brown G (1985) Topic analysis: an objective measure of the consultation and its application to computer assisted consultations. British Medical Journal 290: 1789–91.

Pringle M, Robins S, Brown G (1986) Timer: a new objective measure of consultation content and its application to computer assisted consultations. British Medical Journal 293: 20–2.

Purves I N (1996) Prodigy Interim Report. Newcastle upon Tyne: University of Newcastle, Sowerby Unit for Primary Care Informatics.

Rethans J J, Hoppener P, Wolfs G, Diederiks J (1988) Do personal computers make doctors less personal? British Medical Journal 296: 1446–8.

Richards H, Sullivan F M (1996) Computer Use by General Practitioners in Scotland. Report to the Primary Care Development Fund by the Department of General Practice, University of Glasgow.

Ridsdale L, Hudd S (1994) Computers in the consultation: the patient's view. British Journal of General Practice 44: 367–9.

Roland M O, Zander L I, Evans M, Morris R, Savage R A (1985) Evaluation of a computer assisted repeat prescribing programme in a general practice. British Medical Journal 291: 456–8.

Royal College of General Practitioners (1980) Computers in Primary Care. Report of the Computer Working Party. Occasional Paper No. 13. London: RCGP.

Ryan M P (1989) A system for general practice computing in Scotland. Health Bulletin 47(3): 110–19.

Sackett D L, Richardson W S, Rosenberg W, Haines R B (1997) Evidence-Based Medicine – How to Teach and Practice EBM. Edinburgh: Churchill Livingstone.

Scottish Office (1997) Designed to Care. Edinburgh: HMSO.

Secretary of State for Health (1997) The New NHS. London: HMSO.

Sibley J C, Sackett D L, Neufield V, Gerrard B, Rudnick K V, Fraser W (1982) A randomised controlled trial of continuing medical education. New England Journal of Medicine 306: 511–5.

Slawson D C, Shaughnessy A F (1997) Obtaining useful information from evidence based sources. British Medical Journal 314: 947–9.

Solomon G L, Dechter M (1995) Are patients pleased with computer use in the examination room? Journal of Family Practice 41: 241–4.

Sullivan F, Mitchell E (1995) Has general practitioner computing made a difference to patient care? A systematic review of published reports. British Medical Journal 311: 848–52.

Sullivan F M, MacNaughton R J (1996) Evidence used in consultations: interpreted and individualised. Lancet 348: 941–3.

Sullivan F M, Manchip A, Hussain S (1992) Does the arrival of a desk-top computer reduce patients' satisfaction with the consultation in general practice? Theoretical Surgery 7: 454.

Taylor M W, Milne R M, Taylor R J, Duncan R, MacDonald I (1992) The State of General Practice Computing in Scotland and the Characteristics of Computerised Practices: A Survey of 963 Practices. Aberdeen: University of Aberdeen, Department of General Practice.

Tudor Hart J (1992) Rule of halves: implications of increasing diagnosis and reducing dropout for future workload and prescribing costs in primary care. British Journal of General Practice 42: 116–19.

Weingarten M A, Bazel D, Shannon H S (1989) Computerised protocol for preventive medicine: a controlled self-audit in family practice. Family Practice 6(2): 120–4.

Wyatt J, Walton R (1996) Computer based prescribing. Improves decision making and reduces costs. British Medical Journal 311: 1181–2.

Chapter 9
The patient perspective

Patricia Wilkie

Introduction

The society in which patients and doctors live affects the relationship between patients and their doctors as well as between patients and the other professionals who take care of them. In the 17th century, there was the emergence of the new profession of medicine. There are many examples to suggest that the new professional was polite, considerate and almost deferential to his patients, who paid for his services. The 18th and 19th centuries saw the development of modern scientific medicine, with patients slow to accept medical wisdom.

At the beginning of the 20th century, British health care services were provided by several sources. Departments of Public Health, which were the responsibility of local authorities, provided little in the way of personal health care, although individual Medical Officers of Health supported the various voluntary organizations providing infant welfare clinics. The ordinary sick person could seek private medical attention from a general practitioner (GP) if he could afford to pay the minimum official fee of 2s 6d. For the worker earning £1 (20 shillings) per week, this figure was likely to be prohibitive. There were charitable dispensaries, the out-patient departments of voluntary hospitals and, as a last resort, the poor law medical officer. The regularly employed were likely to be members of friendly societies able to call on the services of the 'club' doctor.

The first half of the 20th century was a period when the patient–doctor relationship was characterized by paternalism and an intrinsic confidence and assurance by the medical profession that 'doctor knows best'. The interwar period had not produced a critical patient but instead patients who held the profession in great respect and who were grateful for the treatment and care that they received. It was possibly a very comfortable relationship for both patient and doctor.

The NHS was established in 1948. Patients were to be treated, free at the point of delivery and 'from the cradle to the grave' (Beveridge, 1943). By 1958 there had been an impressive expansion. The number of in-patients treated had increased by a million, waiting lists had been reduced by about 90 000 from a peak in 1950, and urgent and necessary cases were being admitted immediately. Exciting new treatments were being developed. However, it was not until the second half of this century that the emergence of the critical consumer described below was seen and there was a response from government to involve the public, the user, the patient in the health services and in partnership.

The development of consumerism

By the 1960s change was in the air. This was a period during which the consumer voice began to be heard in a way that had not been experienced before; there was a new confidence in the 1960s. Along with 'flower power' and the Beatles, there emerged a new generation that questioned established traditions. This generation had both the ability and the confidence to set up organizations to press for the introduction of change. The emergence of the critical consumer, by no means peculiar to health care, slowly began to change relationships between some patients and their doctors.

In 1964, Gerda Cohen's book *What's Wrong with our Hospitals?* was published. Many were shocked at the author, a journalist who had been prompted to write after a 2-week stay in a gynaecology ward. Cohen attributed many of the failings she described to outdated attitudes on the part of hospital staff and the condescending treatment of patients by doctors. In the same year, Enoch Powell, speaking as Minister of Health, warned hospital staff to beware of the gulf in attitude, outlook, sympathy and comprehension, a gulf that could open up between the inside world of the hospital and the outside world populated by 'peculiar, unreasonable, ungrateful people – patients and their relatives' (Powell, 1985).

Powell had been critical of attitudes in certain maternity hospitals. This was precisely the time when the maternity hospitals were under attack from a new generation of confident mothers who wished to alter the 'conveyor belt' atmosphere of some of these hospitals, who wanted their husbands with them during delivery – a practice that obstetricians and midwives did not encourage – and who wanted to understand what was happening to them. These pressures led to the founding of the Association for the Improvement of Maternity Services (AIMS) and the National Childbirth Trust (NCT). Expectant mothers wanted to be able to be involved as partners in their antenatal care and in the planning of the birth. What seemed logical to women, the patients, was frequently ridiculed by both medical and midwifery staff. Furthermore, from discussions with then members of the NCT, it seems that, at the time, these members assumed that once the ideas of the NCT were accepted by professionals, the job would be finished and the charity dissolved. The NCT continues to be active, pressuring for the implementation of the ideas in *Changing Childbirth* (Department of Health, 1993).

Williamson (1992) suggests that consumer pressure groups are often started from a strong sense of the harmfulness of some institutional or professional practice, and this appears to apply in the case of the following organizations. In 1961, the National Association for the Welfare of Children in Hospital (NAWCH) was founded (its original name being Mother Care for Children in Hospital). The founders were very concerned that the message in the Platt Report of 1959 on *The Welfare of Children in Hospital,* that children needed regular and continuing contact with their parents, was being ignored. NAWCH campaigned and has continued to campaign for the universal adoption of unrestricted visiting in children's wards, for the provision of accommodation to enable mothers to stay in hospital with their children and for better play facilities in children's wards. There was stiff resistance from paediatricians and paediatric ward sisters, who felt that frequent visiting was upsetting for the children and were not impressed by the evidence that purported to show that separation from the mother could give rise to long-term psychological problems. It is a salutary observation that there are today still some paediatric units where the philosophies of NAWCH are not followed.

The Patients' Association was founded in the 1963 following a letter to the *Observer* newspaper from a lady who alleged that she had been the subject of medical experimentation during her pregnancy. The early work of the Patients' Association focused on the patient's right to refuse to be used in the teaching of medical students and the part of the patient in medical research. Since then, the Patients' Association has generalized to focus on lobbying for patients' interests in health care. In recent years, such topics as improved information about medicines and their side-effects have been addressed.

As a result, the Association of the British Pharmaceutical Industry (ABPI) Data Compendium Sheets became available in public libraries in 1990. As discussed later, these documents are fairly indigestible and not necessarily particularly helpful to patients, but at least their public availability was a beginning. What is even more important is that a dialogue had begun between industry, the government, the professions and representatives of patients about the quality of information given to patients about medicines.

In 1974, the Community Health Councils (CHCs) were established to represent the interests of the community in the NHS. There are now many patient and consumer organizations, both statutory and voluntary, related to different aspects of health care. Their number, their variety, their aims and the fact that some are local and some national can be confusing for both consumers and professionals. Organizations have recently grouped themselves into 'umbrella' organizations such as the Long Term Medical Conditions Alliance (LMCA), the Genetics Interest Group (GIG) and the Neurological Alliance, for the purpose of finding joint areas of concern, for more effective lobbying and for communicating the interests of their members.

The patient as consumer

Consumers in the health services are patients or users of health services. Williamson, in an article on a manager's guide to consumerism, suggests that in health care there are three categories of consumer: patients and carers, consumer groups, and consumerists (Williamson, 1995). This classification is helpful for professionals when considering which consumer to consult. Patients and carers are consumers who have a clinical relationship with a practitioner. The views of patients are personal or individual views. Patients do not generally represent the views of other patients simply because they do not know those views.

Consumer groups are usually self-help or other voluntary groups whose aims are to represent the interests of people with specific problems and to lobby on their behalf.

Consumerists are those whose understanding of patients' interests is wider than that of any single organization. Consumerists always put the patient first and often operate at national level. This analysis is also helpful when considering the different roles that patients and consumers of health services have in their interactions with professionals and health care services. Patients can be involved at an individual level, at an organizational level and at a national level.

In the government White Paper *Working for Patients* (Department of Health, 1989a), the NHSME's *Local Voices* (National Health Service Management Executive, 1992) and the Patient's Charter (Department of Health, 1995), there was an increasing emphasis on the patient as a consumer as well as the stated objective of making the services more responsive to consumers. This objective was also enshrined in the 1990 GP contract (Department of Health, 1989b) and in the establishment of medical audit advisory groups (Rees Lewis, 1994) and was quoted by Gaskin (1997). The momentum to consider patients as consumers and to involve them in dialogue with professionals, managers and policy-makers continues.

There are, however, difficulties inherent in the concept of patients as consumers, particularly at the level of the individual patient and the practitioner. Consider, for example, the concept of the 'asymmetry' of information between the practitioner and the consumer or patient described by Williams (1988). The patient consults because the patient requires help and the practitioner has the expertise and knowledge to give help. There is therefore an inherent inequality in the consultation because of the specialist knowledge of the practitioner. However, the patient also comes to the consultation with knowledge of his own situation and his perception of his problem. Take the example of patients with adult polycystic kidney disease. The nephrologist or GP will undoubtedly be concerned with creatinine levels and other tests to indicate how well the kidneys are functioning. However, in one study, patients were most concerned with the symptoms of moodiness, sleepiness, lethargy, headache and back pain and the restrictions that these symptoms placed on their physical activity (Wilkie et al, 1985). The majority of these symptoms are unlikely to appear in medical textbooks, so it was not surprising that many patients were dissatisfied with their out-patient consultation. Neither the patients nor the doctors understood what the other was expecting from the consultation.

The solution was simple. Patients were given information about the condition, about the clinical manifestations, about the tests that would be carried out and the reasons for those tests and about the treatments available. Patients were encouraged to keep a record of their own test results, medication and blood pressure. Where necessary and appropriate, patients took their own blood pressure at home. This exercise resulted in a cohort of highly motivated and knowledgeable patients who, in their own words, felt that they were able to retain some control over their lives even though they had a progressive illness for which there was no cure. They gained a confidence and, with this, an increased willingness to discuss concerns that they had previously felt would have been considered 'silly'. Good working partnerships between patients and their doctors had developed. The medical staff involved in this project reported that they gained in the relationships that they now had with these patients. Patients felt that they had a much greater understanding of their illness and its implications, helping them to plan and adjust their lives accordingly (Wilkie, 1992).

The expectations of modern consumers of health care for information about treatment options, about the benefits and risks of different treatments and about the effectiveness of the different options should help to nurture the partnership between patients and the professionals looking after them and lessen the importance of the asymmetry of information.

The consultation

The consultation is the place where information passes directly from the practitioner to the patient. Most studies about the consultation concern consultations involving doctors and patients rather than other members of the health care team. Medical consultations are rarely characterized by conflict (Martin et al, 1991). Doctors are trained to diagnose and treat diseases and their symptoms. Patients, on the other hand, are concerned with their personal experience of illness. It has already been described how patients may bring to the consultation ideas about their illness and expectations about what can be done for them that differ from the views of the professional. A failure to reconcile these perspectives can give rise to dissatisfaction. Thus the relationship between the doctor and patient may be made uncomfortable if the expectations of the patient are not met. Patients may also have expectations for the outcome of the consultation, such as a prescription, an X-ray or a referral to another specialist, which the doctor does not judge necessary, yet the doctor does not generally explain this to the patient.

There is considerable anecdotal evidence that patients do not find consultations with their GP particularly satisfactory. However, studies such as that of Rashid et al (1989) confirm a high level of patient satisfaction with GPs during the consultation. These investigators also found that, in general, doctors were less satisfied with the consultation than were the patients.

There are several possible reasons why patients may be dissatisfied with the consultation, including that their expectations were not met. In the work by Martin et al (1991), doctors perceived patients to be less ill than patients considered themselves to be. Furthermore, patients saw the cause of their problems to be infection, trauma, stress and social problems, all of which relate to the belief that health is governed mainly by external factors rather than being under the control of the individual. On the other hand, doctors often saw lifestyle factors such as obesity, alcohol and smoking as being the cause of the problem. The authors concluded that there is a wide divergence between doctors and patients about how ill the patient is, and they point to the need for improvement in communication.

In a consultation, it is clear that, because of their professional status and their specialist knowledge, it is not difficult for doctors to retain control of the consultation. The majority of patients are inexperienced in handling the consultation. However, patients do try to get their own way. In a study of parents and ENT doctors, Bloor (1976) found that parents often mentioned the GP's diagnosis and view that the tonsils should be removed rather than directly stating their own opinion that they wished a tonsillectomy for their child. The assumption was that the consultant would be more impressed by the GP's opinion than the parent's and therefore more likely to agree to the operation.

One of the aims of the recent RCGP initiative 'How to work with your doctor' (Royal College of General Practitioners, 1997), which was itself a partnership between doctors and lay people, was to help to redress the 'asymmetry of information' by giving information to patients to enable them to have a more productive relationship with primary health care staff and thereby achieve better health care. In the leaflet 'You and Your GP During the Day' (Royal College of General Practitioners, 1997), recommendations are made about the sorts of topic that the patient may need to consider before the consultation, including:

- when the person first noticed the symptoms or started feeling ill;
- what makes the condition better or worse;
- what the pain or problem actually feels like.

During the consultation, patients can be encouraged to ask:

- What is the cause of the problem?
- How is the problem normally treated?
- What can the patient do about the problem?

- Are there any long-term effects?
- Is there anything that the patient can do to prevent the problem happening again?

Such practical advice should enable the patient to get the most out of the consultation and help both the practitioner and the patient to make the best use of the time available. However, to date, we lack the research evidence to support these aspirations.

Choice

The Patient's Charter (Department of Health, 1995) states that patients have the right to be registered with a GP and to change their GP easily and quickly. There are many questions that consumers may like answered before registering with a practice. It is, however, appreciated that the notion of consumer choice is only meaningful if there is a range of alternatives from which to choose. As Leavey et al (1989) pointed out, whereas there are some 30 000 GPs in the UK, factors such as geography limit that choice for most people to perhaps three or four practices; for those living in rural areas, there may only be one practice available.

The questions that patients as consumers may like answered about a practice include:

- How long in advance do they have to make an appointment to see the doctor of their choice?
- Can patients get advice from a doctor or other professional over the phone?
- What is the practice policy for out-of-hours consultations?
- Is the practice a teaching or training practice?
- Does the practice carry out research?
- Does the practice have personal lists?
- Can patients make appointments with non-medical staff?
- Do patients have to participate in research?
- Can patient have easy access to their medical records?
- Can patients decline to have a medical student present during the consultation?
- Do the doctors have personal lists?
- Does the practice have a patient participation group?

Where can patients get such information? In accordance with the GPs' 'Red Book', which governs standard requirements for practice,

GPs must issue practice leaflets giving information about the range of staff and their qualifications. Information about surgery hours, appointment systems and arrangements for out-of-hours and special clinics offered may also be included in the leaflet. However, practice leaflets still vary considerably in the quality of information offered. Some practices now offer prospective patients the opportunity to speak to a member of the practice team before deciding to join the practice, and it is on such occasions that the above questions can be asked.

There is, however, anecdotal evidence that, even without information, patients do exercise some choice over whom they consult within a practice. Not all patients consult the doctor with whom they are registered even when that doctor is available. Patients learn from their own previous experience or from talking to other patients which doctors in the practice are 'good' for certain problems. Patients can therefore learn which doctor to consult when they want, for example, a prescription quickly without too many questions being asked. Patients also exercise choice by not following or completing a course of treatment (Kasl, 1975). Some patients may simply prefer particular doctors. There is evidence (Kaplan et al, 1989; Horder and Moore, 1990) that the quality of the interaction between doctor and patient can have a major influence on health outcomes. However, in the average consultation time of approximately 7 minutes, considerable skill is required by both doctor and patient to have quality of interaction in the consultation (Marinker, 1997).

Patients, as consumers, will be expecting to make choices. We live in a society where we are constantly making choices. Patients can make choices between different types of treatment, between radical or conservative treatment or no treatment at all (Wilkie, 1996). It is understood that making choices about one's own care may, in some circumstances, be extremely difficult and indeed too difficult for some people. Nevertheless, many patients as consumers wish to make choices about their treatment and care, and to be involved in the decision-making process. To do so, they need information. Moreover, better-informed patients are able to make choices and ask for choice. However, we need to remember that these choices may not be the choice made by the medical profession or by the government. For example, the tendency is for GPs to practise in group practices and in health centres, with some of the doctors offering specialist services. But is this what the patients want? From their research, Baker and Streatfield (1995) concluded that 'patients in this study preferred smaller practices such as supported by members of the Small

Practices Association (SPA), non-training practices and practices that had personal list systems. Practice organisation should be reviewed in order to ensure that the trend towards larger practices that provide a wide variety of services does not lead to a decline in patient satisfaction'. It would appear that many patients are increasingly expecting personal care that reflects a quality of relationship between doctors and their patients, a relationship that must surely be attractive to many practitioners.

It is clear that, if consumers have the motivation to exercise choice and a range of alternatives from which to choose, they then require adequate information about these alternatives. In order to make these choices, they need evidence about treatment options, outcomes, safety and the results of audit. Armed with these sets of information, patients can make informed decisions about their own health (Wilkie, 1996).

Choice in treatment: evidence-based treatment

When patients enter a research project, they normally receive, and certainly ought to receive, a great deal of information about the underlying problem and the treatments being offered in the study. Indeed, it is not considered ethical for patients to be entered into such studies or drug trials without first giving informed consent based on considerable information. This is good patient care and should be part of normal clinical practice.

Neuberger (1994) suggests that what the patient will be considering is:

- information about the aims of the available treatments;
- what the outcome would be without treatments;
- the objective effectiveness of each treatment;
- the alternative treatments;
- what treatment targets will be set;
- the most common side-effects or interactions;
- when one should stop, change or switch treatment;
- whether it is cheaper to prescribe privately or buy over the counter;
- where the doctor got his information about the medicine;
- whether the doctor would use the same information for his family.

Many of these questions are to do with evidence. In the late 1970s, the late Dr Archie Cochrane drew attention to the apparent ignorance of the medical profession about which treatments work effectively. The Cochrane Collaboration, established in 1992 in his memory in response to that challenge, may be one way in which consumers are going to learn what works and what does not work. The Cochrane Centre supports 'the commitment to informed choice for people using health services' and believes that 'there is an urgent need for patients to be provided with information about the effectiveness of health care'. The Centre suggests that this information 'may come from health professionals, through public libraries and increasingly from consumer health information services.' (Cochrane Collaboration, 1993). The Cochrane Collaboration has been running critical appraisal skills programmes (Critical Appraisal Skills Programme, 1995) for consumers and members of consumer groups to enable people to weigh up the evidence of research to see how useful it is for decisions about health care. Consumer groups are gradually acquiring information about the effectiveness of different treatment options and are able to disseminate that information to their members. However, it still remains difficult for individual patients who are not members of such organizations to acquire information about evidence-based medicine.

Choice in treatment: benefits and risks

Patients, as consumers, are increasingly expecting information about risk versus benefit concerning drugs, as recommended for example by RAD-AR, the International Medical Benefit/Risk Foundation (RAD-AR, 1993). As more powerful drugs are being brought into use and being prescribed by GPs, as more patients on complex therapies are now being looked after in their own homes by members of the primary health care team and as more older people are on multiple drug regimes, information about risk versus benefit becomes increasingly important. The need for GPs, nurses in the primary health care team and pharmacists to give patients information about the benefits and risks of medicines has never been greater. This requires having the information to give to patients, being able to communicate appropriately with the patient and also communicating between different members of the team to ensure that consistent information is given to the patient. The information about benefits and risks should always be conveyed in common language. The usefulness even of ordinary words such as 'rare', 'frequent', 'severe' and 'serious', often used to describe the risks of treatments, or of no treatment, need to be carefully considered and evaluated. Information about benefits and risks needs to be balanced to include information about the benefits of the treatment in both the short and the long term, the risks of the treatment and the option of no treatment. Only then can a patient make an informed decision.

Patients expect to have much more information about medicines, what they might interact with and their side-effects (Wilkie, 1995). The ABPI DATA Compendium Sheets are available in public libraries, but this is not well publicized. Even if the public were aware, this source of information is not very user friendly and is therefore unlikely to be of use to most patients. In order to make use of the sheets, the reader first needs to know the name of the drug company as the information is classified by manufacturer. A similar problem exists with the ABPI Compendium of Patient Information Leaflets (Association of the British Pharmaceutical Industry, 1995), which is a list of the patient information leaflets that are enclosed with prescription medicines, but again the Compendium is classified by drug company. Technical information about medicines is increasingly available on the Internet, but the information may not be applicable or appropriate to the individual patient. It is therefore important to consider both the different methods of giving patients information, including reading material, cassettes and interactive videos, and where the information can be made available.

Again with regard to drug treatment, regulations implementing EC directive 92/27/EEC on product labelling and package leaflets came into force on 1 January 1994 and required all newly licenced medicines to have patient information leaflets from that date. For all other products, leaflets are required at the time of the 5-yearly licence renewal. Directive 92/27/EEC sets out the minimum requirements on information to be contained on both the outer and immediate packaging. Unfortunately, most patients do not have an opportunity to read this information until after they have collected the medicines from the pharmacist. We are all aware of the difficulty of absorbing and retaining complex information given in a relatively short consultation. So, even if the prescribing doctor had given information about the drug, not all patients would remember the information. The information available in the patient information leaflet is available in the ABPI Compendium (Association of the British Pharmaceutical Industry, 1995). This book should be available in pharmacies, clinics and surgeries for patients to consult. It can also be used for doctors, nurses, pharmacists and the patient to discuss the proposed drug therapy.

Choice in referral

Patients as consumers now expect to find out which unit, department or hospital has the best results for specific problems. Patients will also be expecting information about how health services work in their area, including information about waiting lists. To some extent, the former information is already available through the publication by the NHSE of league tables in *Patient's Charter News*, through the figures published by different health authorities, through patient disease-specific organizations and through the work of the Cochrane Collaboration. However, this information may not always reach the individual patient who has been told of their need for a particular intervention. Many patients will not have ready access to information produced by their own health authority or any other health authority. They may not be aware that such information exists. Not all patients are members of disease organizations. Furthermore, although 'money is meant to follow the patient' in the new NHS, the reality for most patients is that they will be referred to the unit where the contract is held. As commissioners are currently very keen to reduce the number of extracontractual referrals, and this reduces choice for patients, the patient must be satisfied that the local service is providing the 'best' care.

An article in *Good Housekeeping* magazine (1996) discussed how to find a good gynaecologist. The article recommended that the following questions be asked:

- How many of the particular operations does the gynaecologist perform each year? (The article recommends that it should be 100.)
- What is the complication rate?
- What special training has the gynaecologist had? (Readers are told that the certificate of endoscopic surgery shows expertise in keyhole surgery.)
- Who will carry out the operation? (Readers are instructed to write the name on the consent form.)

This magazine article demonstrates clearly how some patients, as consumers, are now approaching a consultation. If health practitioners want to maintain good relationships between themselves and patients, they need to take these points on board.

Audit

The document *Working for Patients* (Department of Health, 1989a) said that, in future, all doctors were to adopt medical audit in their routine clinical practice. (In 1993, clinical audit became the new requirement and the term 'medical audit' became obsolete.) For many doctors, this merely formalized what they had been doing for a long time in the process of informal clinical review. For clinical audit to be meaningful, the views of the users should be included (Joule, 1992). The report of the Clinical Audit Working Group of the Clinical Outcomes Group (Department of Health, 1994) supported this view and cited the following reasons:

- to keep clinicians focused on their ultimate goal of caring for patients;
- to enable users to share in the responsibilities for decisions about their health;
- because users' views on the performance of clinicians are important and can lead to an improved quality of care;
- because the process of clinical audit should be made accessible to users, as part of a process of public accountability;
- because the criteria for measurement of the effectiveness of services should reflect the values of users.

In primary health care, ways need to be found of involving users, of assessing the views of users, of incorporating their views in the audit process and of disseminating the findings to users. This process has begun (see section on patient participation groups below) but has still to be fully developed. The form that participation should take and the extent to which patients wish to participate in their health care have been the subjects of many papers (for a review, see Brearley, 1990).

Patient choice and health outcomes

The increasing number of chronically ill people in our population has perhaps served as an impetus for the promotion of greater patient participation in health care (Brearley, 1990). Chronic conditions such as hypertension appear to lend themselves to mutual management strategies, as the patient can provide important information to aid management. This seems appropriate since such patients regularly conduct self-management activities. The patient will naturally choose the regime that best fits his lifestyle (Cameron and Gregor, 1987). The health professional's role will be to help the patient to help himself (Connelly, 1987).

Giving patients a more active role in the planning and delivery of health care can have important health benefits. The perception that one has been able to choose to take a more active role may, in itself, enhance the patient's overall sense of well-being (Smith et al, 1984). It was recently stated that 'choice [may] affect outcome via belief in the particular attributable consequences of that choice' (McPherson, 1993). Schulman (1979) demonstrated, in a randomized trial, that successful blood pressure control correlated with the extent to which patients felt they had participated in planning the management of their condition. In a descriptive study (Legg-England and Evans, 1992), subjects at a cardiovascular risk management clinic with higher perceived control over treatment decisions had lower blood pressure than those with lower perceived control. Kee (1996) has also reviewed supportive evidence. He concluded that 'Involving patients more in making therapeutic choices is justified if the doctor can present options in an unbiased and effective manner and if the process improves the outcome of the care delivered.'

Communication

More than 30 years ago, in Cartwright's research, published in the monograph *Human Relations and Hospital Care* (Cartwright, 1964), 60% of patients interviewed mentioned some failure in communication. Recently, Stewart (1995) systematically reviewed studies of patient–physician communication and concluded that effective communication was often positively associated with improved patient health outcomes – physical, emotional and functional. Failures in communication remain and are possibly the most important cause of difficulties in the relationship between doctors and their patients. Communication problems are the most common cause of dissatisfaction and complaints made to Community Health Councils, voluntary organizations, health authorities and Trusts. In 1991, the Health Service Commissioner stated, as quoted in *Improving Communications Between Doctors and Patients*: 'If only communications among members of staff, or with patients were better, there would be a marked reduction in the number of complaints I receive about care provided by the NHS' (Royal College of Physicians, 1997).

Many studies (e.g. Tuckett et al, 1985) that have examined communications between patients and doctors have shown that:

- patients often do not know the meanings of words used by clinicians;
- patients often have their own ideas about illnesses, and these often differ from the orthodox ideas;
- patients often fail to understand what they are told by health care professionals.

Professionals use technical language and may have great difficulty in thinking how these technical words may be explained to the patient. Medical terms such as 'venous cannulation' and 'serial bloods' are unlikely to be familiar to the majority of patients, many of whom have a very hazy idea of their own anatomy, least of all the names and positions of major organs.

The tone and manner in which the information is given are important. Few patients address their doctor in the manner in which they are spoken to. The instruction 'Now I want you to take these tablets three times a day' is not matched by a patient stating 'Now I want you to examine me and prescribe something appropriate', at least not usually! Patients do make more demanding statements that are direct and firm in tone, for example 'Can't anything be done for it, then?' or 'Can I have a sick note for work?', but these are usually of an inquiring nature rather than instructive or evaluative. Consider the female patient who described herself as being generally reluctant to take medicines and felt that her doctor tended to over-prescribe. She phrased her question to the doctor when he gave her a prescription as follows: 'Are those tablets really necessary doctor? Because if not, I'd rather not take them if it will clear up anyway.' The patient is not openly critical but tactfully pivots the doubt back on herself.

The choice of ordinary words used in a clinical setting is also important in giving a particular impression to patients. Consider the use of words used to describe cancer, as discussed in Sonntag's book *Illness as Metaphor* (Sonntag, 1983). Sonntag suggests that the most common metaphors used to describe cancer are drawn from the language of warfare. Cancer cells do not simply multiply: they are invasive. Malignant tumours invade even when they grow slowly. Cancer cells colonize from the original tumour, tumour invasion often continues, and rogue cells will eventually regroup and mount a new assault on the organism. Treatment, too, according to Sonntag, has a military flavour. Radiotherapy uses the metaphors of aerial warfare, patients being bombarded with toxic rays. Treatment aims to kill cancer cells. These words may help some patients, but they are emotive.

When such differences in beliefs exist, and when words with ambiguous meanings are used, it is not surprising that patients often fail to understand what they are told by health care professionals. Consider the recently diagnosed diabetic patient observed by an off-duty nurse. The patient was tucking in to a very large meal inappropriate for her condition. The nurse spoke to her; the patient explained that she was enjoying her lunch – she had had her diet in the morning! Successful patient management depends not only on the quality of communication between the individual patient and the practitioner, but also on good communication between the different members of the primary health care team. Without such interaction between staff, patients may receive conflicting advice and opinion or even be mismanaged.

The potential influence of patients as consumers at the individual level and within the consultation has already been discussed. At a national level, there are increasing examples of the involvement of patients as consumers in the preparation of policy with the NHSE supporting 'greater voice and influence to users of NHS services and their carers in their own care, the development and definition of standards set for NHS services locally and the development of NHS policy both locally and nationally' (Department of Health, 1996). For example, Southampton Community Health Services NHS Trust has produced a local mental health charter reflecting the needs of local people. The charter was produced in collaboration with local patients and their representatives.

Another form of initiative is the formation of a Patient Liaison Group at the Royal College of General Practitioners, an initiative that is now being followed by many of the medical Royal Colleges. Such groups, where there is mutual trust and respect between lay and professional members, offer an excellent example for collaboration.

Shared responsibility

Patients, as consumers, are increasingly expecting to share in the responsibility for their own treatment and health. Some patients, for example patients on maintenance dialysis, diabetics and those with some other chronic disorders, have always done so. However, we have come through a period of paternalistic medicine that has not encouraged patients to think or to be involved in decisions about their own health. Thus there are still patients, particularly older patients, who are not interested in sharing responsibility. There will always be some patients who simply want the doctor to decide for them. The success of sharing responsibility and being 'partners in care' depends on the patient having access to information, as has been described. There is also considerable evidence that when patients are involved in the plans for their treatment, they are much more likely to concord with that treatment (Marinker, 1997).

Sharing responsibility is, however, by definition a two-way process. If, for example, patients want a smooth-running appointment system with minimum waiting time, they must make sure that they cancel appointments that they are unable to keep. Professionals must, on the other hand, inform patients when there has been a delay and offer opportunities for another appointment. Similarly, practitioners should ideally inform patients of the reasons why when they are asked to leave a practice, whilst patients should inform a practice when they are leaving.

Sharing responsibility also means listening to the patient. Modern patients expect to be listened to, and more and more patients are expecting to ask detailed questions and therefore receive answers.

Another way in which responsibility can be shared is in the establishment of a patient participation group within a practice. The National Association of Patient Participation (NAPP) was established in 1978 to:

- give doctors and patients the opportunity to meet in order to discuss topics of mutual interest in the practice;
- provide a means for patients to make positive suggestions about the practice and their own health care;
- encourage health education activities within the practice;
- develop self-help projects to meet the needs of fellow patients;
- act as representative groups to attempt to influence the local provision of health and social care.

The establishment of a NAPP group in a practice gives individuals the opportunity to be involved in the planning and implementation of their primary health care and for doctors and other members of the practice to work with patients to that end.

Skill mix

There is some anecdotal evidence that patients are questioning the concept of skill mix. As discussed in Chapter 3, skill mix has been introduced to make the best, most cost-effective use of the different members of the health care team. The public, however, need to be reassured that tasks previously carried out by one profession are now to be carried out by other professionals with different and possibly 'lesser' qualifications. How do the public learn that certain investigations in, for example, the X-ray department of a community hospital may no longer be carried out by a radiologist but by a radiographer? Indeed, when this happens, are they informed? There is some evidence that patients are happy to be seen by nurses, rather than doctors, for certain procedures. Whilst little is known of the views of consumers about skill mix, it is possible that some members of the public may be sceptical of skill mix, believing that it is merely a cheaper way of producing a poorer service. It may not be, but it is an area that should be discussed with patients and members of the health care team.

Conclusion

General practice and the work of the primary health care team offer a unique service highly valued by the general public. However, a strong working relationship between practitioners, patients and their representatives must be developed to safeguard the service. The following should be considered:

1. Communication between doctors and patients at a national, local and personal level must continue to improve.
2. Consumerism must be accepted. We live in a society in which there are consumer groups representing many and diverse interests. These groups are knowledgeable and articulate, and must be listened to.
3. Co-operation. There needs to be better co-operation between patient representatives and groups of practitioners about such issues as treatment plans, advice and information to be given to patients.
4. Members of the health care team need to learn to cope, within the professional–patient relationship, with well-informed, confident and articulate patients. Patients will increasingly have access to information, for example on the Internet, as well as to scientific literature previously enjoyed solely by the professionals.

The challenge is considerable. The process has already begun.

References

Association of the British Pharmaceutical Industry (1995) Compendium of Patient Information Leaflets 1995–6. London: Datapharm Publications.

Baker R, Streatfield J (1995) What types of general practice do patients prefer? Exploration of practice characteristics influencing patient satisfaction. British Journal of General Practice 45: 654–9.

Beveridge, Sir W (1943) Social Insurance and Allied Services. Cmnd 6404. London: HMSO.

Bloor M (1976) Bishop Berkeley and the adenotonsilectomy enigma. Sociology 10: 44–61.

Brearley S (1990) Patient Participation. The Literature. London: Scutari Press.

Cameron K, Gregor F (1987) Chronic illness and compliance. Journal of Advanced Nursing 12: 671–6.

Cartwright A (1964) Human Relations and Hospital Care. Oxford: Routledge & Kegan Paul.

Cochrane Collaboration (1993) Preparing, Maintaining and Disseminating Systematic Reviews of the Effects of Health Care. Oxford: UK Cochrane Centre.

Cohen G (1964) What's Wrong with our Hospitals? London: Penguin.

Connelly C E (1987) Self care and the chronically ill patient. Nursing Clinics of North America 22: 621–9.

Critical Appraisal Skills Programme (1995) Report to the King's Fund Development Centre. London: CASP.

Department of Health (1989a) Working for Patients. Cmnd 555. London: HMSO.

Department of Health (1989b) General Practice in the National Health Service. The 1990 Contract. London: HMSO.

Department of Health (1993) Changing Childbirth: Part 1: Report of the Expert Maternity Group. London: HMSO.

Department of Health (1994) Clinical Audit in Primary Health Care. Primary Health Care Clinical Audit Working Group of Clinical Outcomes Group. London: HMSO.

Department of Health (1995) The Patient's Charter and You. London: HMSO.

Department of Health (1996) EL(96) 45; Priorities and Planning Guidelines 1997/98. London: HMSO.

Gaskin K (1997) How to Work with Your Doctor: Report of the Royal College of General Practitioners' Patients Liaison Group. London: RCGP.

Good Housekeeping (1996) Good gynae guide. (May): 148.

Horder J, Moore G T (1990) The consultation and health outcomes. British Journal of General Practice 40: 442–3.

Joule N (1992) User Involvement in Medical Audit. London: Greater London Association of Community Health Councils.

Kaplan S H, Greenfield S, Ware J E (1989) Assessing the effects of physician–patient interactions on the outcomes of chronic disease. Medical Care 27(3) (supplement): 110–27.

Kasl S W (1975) Issues in patient adherence to health care regimes. Journal of Human Stress (September): 5–17.

Kee F (1996) Patients prerogatives and perceptions of benefit. British Medical Journal 312: 958–60.

Leavey R, Wilkin D, Metcalfe D H H (1989) Consumerism and general practice. British Medical Journal 298: 737–9.

Legg-England S, Evans J (1992) Patients' choices and perceptions after an invitation to participate in treatment decisions. Social Sciences and Medicine 34: 1217–25.

McPherson K (1993) The best and the enemy of the good: randomised controlled trials, uncertainty and assessing the role of patient choice in medical decision making. Journal of Epidemiology and Community Health 48: 6–15.

Marinker M (1997) From Compliance to Concordance: Achieving Shared Goals in Medicine Taking. London: Royal Pharmaceutical Society/Merck Sharp & Dohme.

Martin E, Russell D, Goodwin S et al (1991) Why patients consult and what happens when they do. British Medical Journal 303: 289–92.

National Health Service Management Executive (1992) Local Voices. Leeds: NHSE.

Neuberger J (1994) Availability of information in an open society. In Marinker M (Ed.) Controversies in health care policies. British Medical Journal 309: 27–41.

The Platt Report (1959) The Welfare of Children in Hospital. London: HMSO.

Powell J E (1985) Medicine and Politics: 1975 and After. London: Pitman Medical.

RAD-AR (International Medical Benefit/Risk Foundation) (1993) Improving Patient Information and Education on Medicines. Report from the Foundation's Committee on Patient Information. Switzerland: RAD-AR.

Rashid A, Forman W, Jagger C, Mann R (1989) Consultations in general practice: a comparison of patients' and doctors' satisfaction. British Medical Journal 299: 1015–16.

Rees Lewis J (1994) Patient view on quality care in general practice: literature review. Social Science and Medicine 39: 655–70.

Royal College of General Practitioners (1997) How to Work with Your Doctor During the Day. London: RCGP.

Royal College of Physicians (1997) Improving Communications Between Doctors and Patients (quoting the London Health Service Commissioner, 1991, Third Report for session 1990–91). London: RCP.

Schulman B A (1979) Active patient orientation and outcomes in hypertension treatment. Medical Care 17: 267–80.

Smith R A, Wallston B S, Forsberg P R, King J E (1984) Measuring desire for control of health care processes. Journal of Personality and Social Psychology 47: 415–26.

Sonntag S (1983) Illness as Metaphor. London: Penguin.

Stewart M (1995) Effective physician–patient communication and health outcomes: a review. Canadian Medical Association Journal 152: 1423–33.

Tuckett D, Boulton M, Olson C, Williams A (1985) Meetings Between

Experts: An Approach to Sharing Ideas in Medical Consultation. London: Tavistock.

Wilkie P (1992) Genetic Counselling and Adult Polycystic Kidney Disease: Patients' Knowledge, Perception and Understanding. PhD Thesis, University of Stirling.

Wilkie P (1995) PILS and information for patients about medicines: a patient's perspective. In Medicines and Patient Information. EPLC Pharma Law Report No. 15, April 1995.

Wilkie P (1996) The expectations of the modern patient. Proceedings of the Royal College of Physicians of Edinburgh 26: 576–80.

Wilkie P, Markova I, Forbes C D, Kennedy A (1985) Consumers' attitudes to genetic counselling in adult polycystic kidney disease. International Journal of Rehabilitation Research 8: 473–7.

Williams A (1988) Priority setting in public and private health: a guide through the ideological jungle. Journal of Health Economics 7: 173–83.

Williamson C (1992) Whose standards? Consumer and Professional Standards in Health Care. Buckingham: Open University Press.

Williamson C (1995) A manager's guide to consumers. Health Service Journal (30 November): 28–9.

Chapter 10
Education for working in the 'new' NHS

Jane Sims

Introduction

Most patient contact with the NHS occurs in primary care settings. Primary care's generalist function enables the provision of a comprehensive, accessible service. The initial chapters of this book serve to highlight the dynamic nature of the NHS, particularly over the past decade. This scenario is likely to continue, not least given the recent change in government. With services in a continual state of flux, health professionals need to adopt a flexible approach. Professional power bases will be tested in the drift from competition to collaboration, from working within professional boundaries to working in partnership. Both inter- and intraprofessional scepticism must be removed to improve shared care. Throughout this book, several authors have emphasized the importance of education, in one shape or another, for the preparation and development of professional skills. Given the shifting sands, what firm foundation is required in contemporary education? This final chapter seeks to address this question.

What academic knowledge base is required to work in the modern NHS? To the fore are biomedicine and social sciences, which broadly encompass some of the other disciplines highlighted in this book: ethics, social policy, psychology, management, public health and epidemiology. Other areas that impact on primary health care services are law and economics. The biomedical approach continues to dominate, but the call for patient-centred care, referred to throughout this book, means that more holistic models are required to respond to consumerism, decentralization and deregulation. Although Kuhn's theory of how scientific beliefs evolve when existing theories fail to explain new problems may not have explicitly guided this paradigm shift, it has none the less occurred (McWhinney, 1983).

This chapter provides an overview of one area of education, that of the GP, in order to consider how learning needs are being met.

The role of the GP

The nature, status and purpose of the GP are changing, particularly as other health professions develop. More than ever, today's GP needs to have broad-based competencies in order to maintain an acceptable performance (Irvine, 1993). In order to determine what the requirements of GP education are, we first need to review the role of the GP. Medical historians have analysed the nature and aim of general practice and considered the factors that have moulded general practice. The intention here is to give an overview of the past and to contemplate the future.

The UK GP's job description is sufficiently loose to allow flexible and individual interpretation. According to the 1974 Leeuwenhorst Working Party of European GPs (Royal College of General Practitioners, 1978, 1995), the GP's main aim is to make an early diagnosis. In her monograph, Heath (1995) gives two much broader roles for the GP: interpreting illness and taking action where there is disease, and acting as a witness to the patient's experience of illness. The doctor helps the patient to understand his illness – the hermeneutic role – and whittles out where there may be disease present. Tudor Hart's (1994) model views the consultation as 'a meeting between experts'.

The GP needs to gather information to interpret the patient's story in the context of social, psychological and economic factors, and to ascribe meaning against the background of a scientific, biomedical model. Listening is a vital skill in assisting patients to make sense of their illness (Williams and Wood, 1986; Toon, 1994). For this, a distinction between illness and disease is required. This has been extensively discussed in the literature (Helman, 1990) and will not be pursued here. Suffice it to say that illness is a subjective state (what the patient presents with) and disease is an objective state (what he leaves with). What the patient brings to the consultation is often poorly defined; the doctor needs to make sense of this in order to proceed. The patient may bring to the consultation many issues that fall well outside the biomedical model – the whole gamut of human existence, distress and suffering. The social sciences would seem a useful adjunct, along with the skills of anthropology and biography. The humanities could assist in broadening communication with patients, enabling clarification of the patient's experience (Midgeley, 1992; Sweeney, 1998). Add to these an understanding of philosophy and a political bent, and the GP's portfolio would be more rounded. To quote Gillon (1997):

> The science of medicine must, if it is to optimise achievement of its objective of improving the practice of healthcare, collaborate with the art of medicine, a central part of which is understanding of people.

The GP's role also involves empathy, which can be established during the long-term relationship between patient and GP. Rudebeck (1992) cites empathy as a core skill of general practice that assists in validating the patient's illness experience. Taylor (1997) has recently commented that the element of compassion is being eroded in the newer, short-term approach to care delivery. In an age of short-termism, continuity of care can aid growth of understanding and enrich practice (Wynne-Jones, 1993). The need for a patient-centred (Levenstein et al, 1986; Stewart et al, 1995) approach is vital.

There are a number of models of practice for the GP, although it is unlikely that any individual GP fits any one particular model. The traditional paradigm is the biomechanical or Oslerian model. In this model, the doctor acts like a bio-engineer, healing by the application of biological science. Other models have tended to emerge to address the inadequacies of the 'establishment' biomedical model for medical practice (Seedhouse, 1991). Toon (1994) has discussed the place of the teleological, humanist model; such models include the hermeneutic model, best exemplified by the work of Balint and his followers (Balint, 1964). A third type is the preventive, public health model, such as the anticipatory care model espoused by Tudor Hart (1988).

A cautionary note should be sounded at this point. Whilst these models have allegiances to existing philosophies and concepts, they evolved experientially, often with a political impetus, rather than being derived from any existing theoretical basis. The models propose different views of what the doctor–patient relationship should entail and of its founding principles. Either implicit or explicit in the models is an ethical viewpoint; a moral stance regarding justice is also incorporated. To quote Toon (1994):

> despite its lack of an articulated coherent philosophical basis, general practice has flourished as a profession and an academic field for many decades.

The scope of general practice has broadened with the accessibility of a wider range of investigations and the availability of technology to aid therapeutics. In addition to the potential responsibilities of hospital-at-home patients, Fulop in Chapter 7 highlighted aspects of the GP's extended role in areas such as minor surgery and minor injuries units. Gordon in Chapter 1 highlighted the benefits of the gate-keeper role, which allowed general practice to develop during the latter half of the 20th century. However, both she and Meads (Chapter 2) note that independent practitioner status, and to a degree fundholding, created inappropriate variations in service provision although these have been remedied somewhat in recent years, for example via accountability under the 1990 contract and continuing medical education. Thus the role of the GP is gradually changing, from that of gate-keeper to that of both purchaser and provider of services. GPs need to be involved in discussions of new extended roles, since politicians and planners are not always *au fait* with the discipline (Metcalfe, 1992).

Through the internal market of the Conservative years, many GPs emerged as purchasers and had to address public/community health as well as individual needs. This trend will continue as more GPs (and nurses) become involved in locality commissioning groups. As GPs increase their involvement in commissioning and purchasing secondary care, the traditional power base of the consultant is being eroded, some would say for the better. The GP is increasingly having to consider a public as well as a personal health perspective (Fry and Horder, 1994). There are opportunities for greater links and the merging of skills with public health physicians. This may lead to the obsolescence of the 1990 GP contract, with its core general medical services, as an extended range of services are being provided within primary care and a new means of assessing ability to deliver is required.

However, Heath (1995) argues that GPs must not lose patient trust by involvement in health rationing decisions, which act in opposition to the GPs' role of patient advocate and their partisanship. Market values have cast the patient in the role of consumer (see Chapter 9) with rising expectations, whilst a cash-limited NHS means that the GP has fewer resources to meet their needs. Heath comments on the incongruity of individual consumer gratification in this social context and quotes McWhinney, who noted the danger of GPs becoming 'purveyors of a commodity rather than members of a vocational profession providing a public service'.

GP education

A doctor should have at least one other way of thinking than that of the doctor, one other system of mental discipline than that of medicine. (Charlton, 1993)

Biological theories, in which functional disturbances create disease, have dominated medical education. Social theories, in which social influences upon health maintenance are highlighted, have been marginalized (Swanson, 1984). Medical education at all stages is still based upon the biomedical model. As a result, traditional education has involved the acquisition of a scientific but uncritical knowledge base (Horrobin, 1978). Over the years, a knowledge of people, their psychosocial context and how to communicate with people has been sidelined in favour of a skills, task-based route to clinical competency. Rebscher (1993) has commented that:

> the social obligation of medicine is not limited to the application of technical-curative methods. It rather also encompasses prevention, rehabilitation as well as co-operation with other health professionals. Furthermore, medicine is tied into a social, economical and legal framework which has a direct impact on medical practice. Training in social medicine in medical education has to address these relationships.

Sociology input enables doctors to understand social factors, for example values and norms, that influence and predict behaviour. Pendleton et al (1989) emphasized that these variables influence not only the initial visit to the doctor, but also the outcome of healing. From an educational perspective, it has been found to be useful to expose students to this learning early in their training and to allow for its application via practical experience: skills and an understanding of their importance can develop concurrently (Ojanlatva et al, 1995).

Objectivity versus subjectivity

Whereas biosciences focus on objectivity, social sciences emphasize the importance of subjectivity. In arguing for a more humanistic, person-centred approach to health care, Doran (1983) suggests that:

> The entrenchment of the disease model in medical education is a direct and inevitable result of the entrenchment of scientific method in medicine, to the point where such method is ideologically accepted in medical practice.

Whilst medicine has been swayed by the authoritativeness of scientific objectivity, medicine undoubtedly contains much subjectivity, particularly in primary care practice. Doctors' judgements have both empirical and evaluative components, as exemplified by the classification of medicine as both an art and a science. Pendleton (1995) has drawn attention to the lack of a supporting base for non-clinical decision-making in the profession:

> The [young] doctor needs to acquire the skills to work with ethical and other dilemmas, the fortitude to live with uncertainty and the judgement to manage the competing demands of the health authority, community, patients, practice partners and family.

Boorse (1975) stated that primary care medicine is seen as more value laden than hospital medicine and that this led to its lower status in the past. GPs need to be able to tolerate uncertainty and ambiguity, to fill the gap between a curative and a palliative model of care (Sweeney, 1998).

Fulford (1993) has posited a 'bridge theory of illness' that bonds medical and social theories into 'an integrated picture of the conceptual structure of medicine as a whole'. Illness is found between health and disease. Here, illness maintains its value-laden, experiential nature and is seen as 'action failure' (Nordenfelt, 1987), and the patient's perspective of value is given full credence. As stated earlier, the primary care practitioner has a crucial evaluative role in distinguishing between illness and disease. In a bridge theory, health care is no longer reliant upon the opinion of one expert but can use the multiple expertise of a team. Fulford confirms the practical relevance of a bridge theory by analysing its use in guiding the Oxford Practice Skills Project (Hope and Fulford, 1994). This aims to integrate ethics, law and communication skills – practice skills – with more traditional scientific knowledge during the clinical years to demonstrate their interdependency.

Historical perceptive

Virchow was an early supporter of social science in medicine, and the so-called 'social physician', as were others in the 18th century, such as Frank (Wegar, 1992).

Sigerist was a pre-World War II proponent of the merging of the biological and social sciences to enable the physician to act as an advocate in society and a change agent (Brickman, 1994). A medical historian, he emphasized the use of the social sciences to address contemporary issues, such as inequality in access to health care. Medical care had to be accompanied by social reform. Sigerist foresaw the move towards preventive, 'whole person' medicine and the need for doctors to be suitably equipped for this. He contributed to US medical education reform in the 1930s and 40s by reiterating that medicine is an applied science and by calling for the use of a more broad-based concept of science (Sigerist, 1960). He reminded the establishment of the social context of health care: disease is as often the result of social circumstances as it is pathogenic in origin. Sigerist's model curriculum contained philosophy, ethics, anthropology, economics, social medicine and public health.

In the UK, the importance of the behavioural sciences (psychology, sociology and ethics) in medical education have been widely debated since the Goodenough report (Ministry of Health and Department of Health for Scotland, 1944). The Todd report (Royal Commission on Medical Education, 1968) recommended that such teaching be integral to the curriculum but gave no specific instructions on its aims and content.

There are, however, dissenters. Wegar (1992) views the espousal of social science by US physicians during the 1960s as a means of pacifying society with respect to the profession's commitment to community issues. She is also sceptical of the more recent emphasis on medical ethics. Although it entails a more individual-based approach, Wegar sees the impetus as being economical rather than educational, given the debate on access and the distribution of health care. Given the anxieties of UK GPs over their potential role in rationing health care, such misgivings may also arise here.

Undergraduate medical education

The intimate interaction between doctor and patient that occurs in general practice is not reflected in secondary care, yet undergraduate medical education chiefly consists of teaching for and in that setting. Although acute medicine still takes precedent, modern education has sought to adapt to include more experience of chronic and minor illness. The myth of cure, perhaps more common in secondary care, has to be overcome where necessary, for example for patients with chronic conditions that can be treated but not cured (Tallis, 1994). In addition, the socialization process of medicine allied to the traditional educational package has been difficult to modify: fixative and curative ideals need to be unlearned. Whilst Conrad (1988) has argued that changes to the selection process for intake to medical schools will have greater impact upon doctors' attitudes and behaviour than will the curriculum content, others emphasize the even greater influence of socialization on the prevailing organization of professional practice (Eisenberg, 1988).

Fortunately, the scene is changing. More attachments are occurring in primary care settings to reflect the shift in the balance of care provision. Academic and service GPs have actively supported the developments for more community-based teaching. There are likely to be increased opportunities for community-based education. General practices will provide much input, with members of the primary health care team, including practice managers, acting as an education resource for a variety of students. Medical students need not only to observe how GPs work, but also to gain an appreciation of the roles of other primary health care team members. Students are benefiting from spending more time in the community rather than just in general practices, but in other settings, from mental health units to drug drop-in centres. We have already seen the move towards pre-registration house officer posts in the community.

Undergraduate medical education has undergone major structural curriculum changes during the 1990s following the publication of *Tomorrow's Doctors: Recommendations on Undergraduate Medical Education* (General Medical Council, 1993). The aim was to achieve a greater degree of standardization across courses than had previously existed and to reduce curriculum overload. The curriculum has become systems based, with input from basic scientists and clinicians throughout, thereby removing the existing pre-clinical/clinical divide.

The prescribed framework of the General Medical Council, which is responsible for the register attesting to a doctor's fitness to practice, incorporates goals and objectives for undergraduate medical education that both implicitly and explicitly refer to the importance of non-biomedical constructs in shaping knowledge, skills and attitudes:

The student should acquire a knowledge and understanding of health and its promotion, of disease, its prevention and management, in the context of the whole individual and his or her place in the family and in society. (para 39)

a knowledge and understanding of ... how patients react to illness or to the belief that they are ill, and how illness behaviour varies between social and cultural groups; the environmental and social determinants of disease ... human relationships, individual and community; the importance of communication, both with parents and their relatives and with other professionals ...; ethical and legal issues relevant to the practice of medicine; the organisation, management and provision of health care. (para 40) (General Medical Council, 1993)

Whilst the recommended core themes reflect these objectives and include, for example, communication skills, public health, handicap, disability and rehabilitation, and 'man in society'(psychology and sociology relevant to medicine), there is a variation in the weight given to these topics across medical schools. These topics should ideally run throughout the 5-year course and be integral to any progressive assessment process.

Academic departments of general practice have contributed to these reforms, not only by teaching communication skills, but also by embracing the aims of the new curriculum (Robinson et al, 1994). Medical educationalists have sought to incorporate ethics (Fox et al, 1995), medical history (Lederer et al, 1995) and medical geography (Matthews, 1993) into the undergraduate curriculum. Glasgow University has adopted the General Medical Council's recommendation for arts and humanities to appear in the curriculum and is amongst those universities allowing students to study literature, philosophy and history in special study modules (Downie et al, 1997; Macnaughton, 1997). Even so, not all institutions have embraced such an holistic approach as that of the Oxford Practice Skills Project (Hope and Fulford, 1994). Nor can we assume that interest developed via non-core special study modules will breach the gap. The desire for 'interdisciplinary synthesis' may not have been fulfilled as yet. We need further confirmation that areas such as health psychology, public health, ethics and medical law are being adequately represented in the training of our doctors.

There are some critics of this broader curriculum. Education cannot afford to become so diffuse that doctors are no longer properly trained for their main functions of diagnosis and treatment (Macnaughton, 1998). Wales (1978) has questioned teaching behavioural sciences to doctors if they face time pressures which mean that they cannot put these skills into practice. However, doctors need to be able to identify psychosocial needs in order to refer patients on. Gropper (1987) demonstrated that whilst US family doctors receive more social science input than other US primary care-based physicians, their psychosocial knowledge is not significantly better. Although his work is methodologically weak, it still provides a salient message regarding the importance that some physicians place on this material. In contrast, a Nigerian study found final-year medical students to be more aware of the importance of social factors as determinants of health and illness than other (arts/social sciences) students (Nnodim and Osuji, 1995).

Models of education

The GMC is currently reviewing the impact of 'Tomorrow's Doctors'. Their reports show examples of good practice (General Medical Council, 1996, 1997). There is certainly evidence of more integrated core curricula, albeit using the more conservative of organizational approaches discussed by Vars (1991). Problems of curriculum overload are also being addressed via more androgogical educational methods (Knowles, 1984) such as problem-based, self-directed and student-centred learning, which encourage context and process-based learning rather than the traditional content-based programmes.

Students are being given more opportunities, from an earlier point in their training, to apply learning in practical situations. For example, Scottish educators report on the various benefits of using a patient interview scheme as a learning tool on a pre-clinical behavioural sciences course (Orbell and Abraham, 1993). Snadden and Yaphe (1996) obtained positive feedback from fourth-year medical students on the opportunity for hands-on practice during general practice attachments. Patients can help students to learn more about the behavioural model of medical practice, having a number of key roles to play. They can often be the most effective tutors, and many medical schools involve patients from the local community in their teaching programmes.

The 21st century may see a wider adoption of the North American model of graduate medical education. Despite scepticism over the suitability of arts graduates for medical training (*Independent*, 1997), a number of medical schools, such as St George's in London, are already pioneering fast-track degrees for graduates.

Post-graduate education for general practice

We have noted the advances being made at undergraduate level, but what about the post-graduate picture? Traditionally, undergraduate and post-graduate teaching have been conducted by separate departments. The gap is closing, one Scottish university having a joint department, and several institutions offering Masters courses. Until recently, London medical schools provided support for the London

Academic Training Scheme, in which recently qualified GPs developed teaching and research skills in academic departments of general practice.

From the introduction in 1979 of legislation requiring vocational training for GP principals (NHS England and Wales, 1979) and mandatory training from 1982, GP post-graduate education took some time to develop today's structure, hindered in part by financial constraints. The RCGP is currently in favour of GP registrars spending 18 months training in the general practice setting. It would also like to see a further period of 2 years' higher professional education for recently qualified GPs. As part of this move, the Vocationally Trained Associates (VTA) scheme was set up in 1994 to provide a second year in general practice before becoming a partner.

Vocational training for GPs is regulated and monitored nationally via the Joint Committee on Postgraduate Training for General Practice (JCPTGP), but it is organized regionally. There is no national curriculum, although all regionally organized courses have a mandate to provide training that will fulfil centrally prescribed summative assessment criteria (Conference of Postgraduate Advisers in General Practice Universities of United Kingdom, 1996). Several regions follow the principles laid down in the RCGP's early publication on learning and teaching in general practice (Royal College of General Practitioners, 1972). Today's GP registrars increasingly obtain experience in community hospitals, health authorities and commissioning agencies to gain, for example, a more public health perspective.

Most would agree that competency to achieve desired organizational and attitudinal ends underpins professional training. Views on the best means of achieving these ends are inevitably fluid. Whilst some means can be empirically tested, few are value free. General practice is based on probabilities rather than certainty. Vocational training therefore takes a very open and flexible approach to meeting educational needs. In general, the emphasis tends to be towards the practical – clinical and administrative skills are learnt – rather than the academic. Where topics from the various disciplines are taught, the onus is likely to be on application rather than theory, although inevitably within such a loose system, there will be exceptions (Mathie, personal communication, 1997).

The registrars' teachers, themselves GPs, are taught educational methodologies, but there is no universal policy that covers their training or its content. Vocational training is an area that has been somewhat difficult to evaluate, given that only broad standards (from the RCGP and JCPTGP) exist against which to compare local training schemes. Several regional schemes have been compared with the Oxford Region system, which laid down specific objectives (Oxford Region Course Organisers and Regional Advisers, 1985) and, by serendipity, have been found to have met these objectives.

Whilst there has been some criticism that the current summative assessment is a test of *minimal* competence (Rhodes and Wolf, 1997), there is little evidence that the system is any less successful than others in producing competent practitioners. Nor should it be overlooked that the post-graduate training of doctors for general practice is probably far more streamlined than that of other areas of medicine. Furthermore, it is encouraging that GP post-graduate education has, albeit intuitively, incorporated problem-centred, independent learning (Marwick, 1989; Neighbour, 1992), an approach that is rapidly gaining credibility in undergraduate education as a progressive and innovative mode of education. Future programmes need to promote a more systematic approach to experiential learning.

For many years, the RCGP and the Association of University Departments of General Practice (AUDGP) have recognized the value of non-biomedical topics (e.g. Association of University Teachers in General Practice, 1984), but the onus has been upon trying to create a more streamlined structure for GP education nationwide. The RCGP has recently produced a blueprint for the college membership examination (MRCGP). This is taken by increasing numbers of GPs. A raised profile is given to the following areas:

- personal care;
- team issues and practice management;
- values and attitudes – ethics, integrity, consistency and caritas;
- self-awareness – insight and reflective learning;
- medico-political, legal and societal issues.

At present, GP registrars commonly sit this exam in addition to the summative assessment that is the end-point of their vocational training. Moves are afoot to combine the two processes into one examination, but, as might be expected, there are political and other considerations to be dealt with.

The extent to which individual GPs espouse these topics in daily practice remains to be seen – this is not easily measured by traditional examination methods.

We should not lose sight of the fact that an adequate knowledge of medicine overall and the skill to apply this knowledge is crucial and must be supported by continuing medical education.

Continuing professional development

Medical education is certainly a dynamic area and it will be several years before we see changes in terms of the attitudes and behaviour of doctors emerging from recent changes in training. It will be via continuing education and training that health professionals will most rapidly contribute to good clinical practice.

At present, individual GPs are expected to participate in continuing education as part of their professional responsibilities: an average of 10 days continuing medical education per year is recommended, for which re-imbursement is available via a post-graduate education allowance. Courses should be validated and provide credit rather than being one-off, unevaluated interventions. Educational programmes need to be relevant: to accommodate for clinical developments, changes in health service organization and changes in patients' expectations. The emphasis should be upon continuing, long-term education. Learning opportunities and outcomes must be linked to professional experience: self-directed learning, using audit and research, is central to continuing medical education (Stanley et al, 1993). Mentorship is being used to facilitate a more participative mode of education. The intended outcome is that practitioners will integrate learning within daily practice.

For the clinical generalist, continuing education is a means of pursuing specialist interests. A number of specialist Masters courses are available throughout the UK, and a number of regions and the RCGP fund clinical and research fellowship schemes to enable GPs to acquire training in areas such as dermatology, gastroenterology and accident and emergency medicine.

The Internet will be increasingly used to develop and maintain knowledge and skills: health professionals are already learning to use these systems, for example Doctor's Desk (De Lusignan, 1997). The benefits of teleconferencing and CAL were highlighted in Chapter 8. Distance learning is set to feature prominently in the future education of busy practitioners.

It is worth noting that there has been some debate about the current mandatory structure for continuing medical education (Bashook and Parboosingh, 1998), and this is likely to continue. In addition to the various social, political and regulatory pressures being exerted, financial pressures will more than ever play a part. It remains to be seen whether a balance can be struck between calls for cost-efficiency on the one hand and innovative, problem-based learning on the other.

The theory of general practice

Whilst the profession has been wrestling to accommodate the revisions imposed by an ever-changing NHS and dealing with the more structural issues of education, the underpinning theory of the discipline has not received the attention it deserves. The study of epistemology concerns the nature of knowledge and the justification of truth. It has been widely applied in other disciplines but has had limited application in the health professions. For example, Howie (1996) comments that there has been a lack of reflection on the theory surrounding clinical decision-making. He suggests that this may partially explain why GPs are finding it difficult to cope with the conflicting demands of increasing patient expectation and clinical capability on one hand and finite, inadequate resources on the other.

The doctor–patient relationship is key to general practice, and the consultation is the main transaction. Whilst the dynamics of the consultation are taught and researched and the skills learnt, the underlying disciplines are not always formally studied or explained in GP training. As a result, much practice is developed experientially, with a focus on intuition rather than theoretical grounding. McWhinney (1996) has said that general practice must become less pragmatic and more theoretical in order to gain acceptance. An integration of the abstract and the particular is required.

McWhinney (1996) also highlighted that general practice is the only medical discipline that is defined in terms of relationships rather than disease and where mind–body dualism is minimized. To this end, GPs tend to think about individual patients in an holistic manner rather than using a mechanistic approach based upon generalized abstractions. GP education needs to reflect this. Murdoch (1997), reflecting upon McWhinney's earlier concerns (McWhinney, 1983), questioned how teaching about models of consultation was to be given when most clinical teaching occurs in hospitals and only 6% of academic posts are in general practice. In referring to this phenomenon as 'Mackenzie's puzzle', he calls for a clarification of the philosophy that underpins general medical practice, teaching and research (Murdoch, 1997).

Educationalists like Mathers and Rowland have argued for the use of post-modern theory to guide education for general practice (Mathers and Rowland, 1997). These authors draw attention to the emphasis that continues to be placed upon the scientific method of defining 'truth'. They believe that general practice would be better understood using post-modern theory, which acknowledges the different perceptions of reality and their influence upon knowledge. Such a theoretical basis would seem to be a better basis for the accommodation of the dynamism and uncertainties of general practice.

Whilst not demeaning the value of the current trend towards evidence-based practice and learning, Ridsdale (1996) has called for a broader approach to acquiring and using knowledge, one that involves the development as well as the testing of theory. Again, this points to the relative scarcity of theories within general practice and primary care. The move towards using qualitative research methodologies to explore the psychosocial aspects of general practice should help to enrich future practice. Schön's work on the reflective practitioner (Schön, 1990) could guide all levels of GP learning, particularly in relation to the consultation (Shapiro and Talbot, 1991). Schön's work has already been promoted in nurse education. The concept of 'grounded theory' (Glaser and Strauss, 1967), in which theory is developed inductively from observations, seems suited to certain elements of general practice. Certainly, general practice would benefit from the development of more specific theories to explain its varied activities.

Conclusion

Finally, we should not forget the importance of patient education, to encourage the rational lifelong consumption of health services. Wilkie has discussed the emerging role of the patient in planning health care in detail in Chapter 9. With changes such as the growing use of OTC medications and consultation with the pharmacist or the nurse about minor ailments, patients are increasingly likely to receive health care and advice from a range of professionals: this will involve some change in attitudes and beliefs. There is also an educational need to alter public perception of the preferred sector for care provision and to 'sell the unpalatable truths of a utilitarian system of resource allocation' (Coulter, 1995). Patients, purchasers and providers all need to be suitably educated to adapt to the NHS of the 21st century.

References

Association of University Teachers in General Practice (1984) Undergraduate Medical Education in General Practice. Occasional Paper No. 28 Exeter: RCGP.

Balint M (1964) The Doctor, his Patient and the Illness, 2nd Edn. London: Pitman Medical.

Bashook P G, Parboosingh J (1998) Recertification and the maintenance of competence. British Medical Journal 316: 545–8.

Boorse C (1975) On the distinction between disease and illness. Philosophy and Public Affairs 5: 49–68.

Brickman J P (1994) Science and the education of physicians: Sigerist's contribution to American medical reform. Journal of Public Health Policy 15: 133–64.

Charlton B (1993) Holistic medicine or the humane doctor. British Journal of General Practice 43: 475–7.

Conference of Postgraduate Advisers in General Practice Universities of United Kingdom (1996) Summative Assessment: General Practice Training. Winchester: National Office for Summative Assessment.

Conrad P (1988) Learning to doctor: reflections on recent accounts of the medical school years. Journal of Health and Social Behaviour 29: 323–32.

Coulter A (1995) Shifting the balance from secondary to primary care: needs investment and cultural change. British Medical Journal 311: 1447–8.

De Lusignan S (1997) What is the Doctor's Desk? General Practice Manager 29: 3–5.

Doran G A (1983) Scientism versus humanism in medical education. Social Science and Medicine 17: 1831–5.

Downie R S, Hendry R A, Macnaughton R J, Smith B H (1997) Humanising medicine: a special study module. Medical Education 31: 276–80.

Eisenberg L (1988) Science in medicine: too much or too little and too limited in scope? American Journal of Medicine 84: 483–91.

Fox E, Arnold R M, Brody B (1995) Medical ethics education: past, present and future. Academic Medicine 70: 761–9.

Fry J, Horder J (1994) Primary Health Care in an International Context. London: Nuffield Provincial Hospitals Trust.

Fulford K W M (1993) Praxis makes perfect: illness as a bridge between biological concepts of disease and social conceptions of health. Theoretical Medicine 14: 305–20.

General Medical Council (1993) Tomorrow's Doctors. Recommendations on Undergraduate Medical Education. Issued by the Education Committee of the General Medical Council in pursuance of section 5 of the Medical Act, 1983. London: GMC.

General Medical Council (1996) Implementation of the 1993 Recommendations on Undergraduate Medical Education: Report of the Informal Visits which Took Place in 1995. London: GMC.

General Medical Council (1997) Implementation of the 1993 Recommendations on Undergraduate Medical Education: Second Report of the Education Committee. London: GMC.

Gillon R (1997) Imagination, literature, medical ethics and medical practice. Journal of Medical Ethics 23: 3–4.

Glaser B G, Strauss A L (1967) The Discovery of Grounded Theory. Chicago: Aldine.

Gropper M (1987) Family medicine and psychosocial knowledge: how many hats can the family doctor wear? Social Science and Medicine 25(11): 1249–55.

Heath I (1995) The Mystery of General Practice. London: Nuffield

Provincial Hospitals Trust.

Helman C G (1990) Culture, Health and Illness, 2nd Edn. London: Wright.

Hope R A, Fulford K W M (1994) Medical education: patients, principles and practice skills. In Gillon R (Ed.) Principles of Health Care Ethics. Oxford: John Wiley & Sons.

Horrobin D (1978) Medical Hubris: A Reply to Ivan Illich. Edinburgh: Churchill Livingstone.

Howie J G R (1996) Addressing the credibility gap in general practice: better theory; more feeling; less strategy. British Journal of General Practice 46: 479–81.

Independent (1997) Wanted: arts graduates with a convincing bedside manner. 27 November, Education Plus, pp. 2–3.

Irvine D H (1993) General practice in the 1990s: a personal view on future developments. British Journal of General Practice 43: 121–5.

Knowles M (1984) Andragogy in Action: Applying Modern Principles of Adult Learning. San Francisco: Jossey-Bass.

Lederer S E, More E S, Howell J D (1995) Medical history in the undergraduate medical curriculum. Academic Medicine 70: 770–6.

Levenstein J, McCracken E, McWhinney I et al (1986) The patient-centred clinical method. 1: A model for the doctor patient interaction in family medicine. Family Practice 3: 75–9.

Macnaughton R J (1997) Special study modules: an opportunity not to be missed. Medical Education 31: 49–51.

Macnaughton R J (1998) Medicine and the arts: let's not forget the medicine. British Journal of General Practice 48: 952–3.

McWhinney I (1983) Changing models: the impact of Kuhn's theory on medicine. Family Practice 1: 3–8.

McWhinney I (1996) The importance of being different. British Journal of General Practice 46: 433–6.

Marwick J (1989) Learner-centred approaches. Journal of the Association of Course Organisers 5: 6–9.

Mathers N, Rowland S (1997) General practice – a post-modern specialty? British Journal of General Practice 47: 177–9.

Matthews S A (1993) Curriculum redevelopment: medical geography and women's health. Journal of Geography in Higher Education 17(2): 91–102.

Metcalfe D (1992) Care in the capital: what needs to be done. British Medical Journal 305: 1141–4.

Midgeley M (1992) Science as Salvation: A Modern Myth and its Meaning. London: Routledge.

Ministry of Health and Department of Health for Scotland (1944) Report of the Interdepartmental Committee on Medical Schools (Goodenough Report). London: HMSO.

Murdoch J C (1997) Mackenzie's puzzle – the cornerstone of teaching and research in general practice. British Journal of General Practice 47: 656–8.

Neighbour R (1992) The Inner Apprentice. Dordrecht: Kluwer Academic.

NHS England and Wales (1979) The National Health Service (Vocational Training) Regulations No. 1644. London: HMSO.

Nnodim J O, Osuji C U (1995) Comparison of medical and non-medical student attitudes to social issues in medicine. Medical Education 29: 273–7.

Nordenfelt L (1987) On the Nature of Health: An Action-theoretic Approach. Dordrecht: Reidel.

Ojanlatva A, Rautava P, Hyssala L et al (1995) Teaching sociology of medicine: the group process. Medical Education 29: 205–10.

Orbell S, Abraham C (1993) Behavioural sciences and the real world: report of a community interview scheme for medical students. Medical Education 27: 218–28.

Oxford Region Course Organisers and Regional Advisers (1985) Priority Objectives for GP Vocational Training. RCGP Occasional Paper No. 30. London: RCGP.

Pendleton D (1995) Professional development in general practice: problems, puzzles and paradigms. British Journal of General Practice 45: 377–81.

Pendleton D, Schofield T, Tate P, Havelock P (1989) The Consultation: An Approach to Learning and Teaching. Oxford: Oxford University Press.

Rebscher H (1993) Developing social medicine competence in medical education – goals in social medicine education for the practising physician from the viewpoint of mandatory public insurance. Gesundheitwesen 55 (supplement 2): 72–4.

Rhodes M, Wolf A (1997) The summative assessment package: a closer look. Education for General Practice 8: 1–7.

Ridsdale L (1996) Evidence-based learning for general practice. British Journal of General Practice 46: 503.

Robinson L A, Spencer J A, Jones R H (1994) Contribution of academic departments of general practice to undergraduate teaching, and their plans for curriculum development. British Journal of General Practice 44: 489–91.

Royal College of General Practitioners (1972) The Future General Practitioner: Learning and Teaching. London: RCGP.

Royal College of General Practitioners (1978) The Work of the General Practitioner. Occasional Paper No. 6. London: RCGP.

Royal College of General Practitioners (1995) The Nature of General Medical Practice. Report from General Practice No. 27. London: RCGP.

Royal Commission on Medical Education (1968) Report of the Royal Commission on Medical Education (Todd Report). Cmnd 3569. London: HMSO.

Rudebeck C E (1992) General practice and the dialogue of clinical practice: on symptoms, symptom presentations and bodily empathy. Scandinavian Journal of Primary Health Care 10(3, supplement 1): 161–2.

Schön D A (1990) Educating the Reflective Practitioner. San Francisco: Jossey-Bass.

Seedhouse D (1991) Liberating Medicine. Chichester: John Wiley & Sons.

Shapiro J, Talbot Y (1991) Applying the concept of the reflective practitioner to understanding and teaching family medicine. Family Medicine 23: 450–6.

Sigerist H E S (1960) Current unrest in the medical world. In Roemer M I (Ed.) Sociology of Medicine. New York: M D Publications.

Snadden D, Yaphe J (1996) General practice and medical education: what do medical students value? Medical Teacher 18: 31–4.

Stanley I, Al-Shehri A, Thomas P (1993) Continuing education for general practice. 1: Experience, competence and the media of self-directed learning for established general practitioners. British Journal of General Practice 43: 210–14.

Stewart M, Brown J B, Weston W W et al (1995) Patient-centred Medicine: Transforming the Clinical Method. Thousand Oaks, CA: Sage.

Swanson A G (1984) Medical education in the United States and Canada. Physicians for the 21st century: report of the project panel on the general professional education of the physician and college preparation for medicine (Muller S et al, Eds). Journal of Medical Education 59(2): 35–42.

Sweeney B (1998) The place of the humanities in the education of a doctor. British Journal of General Practice 48: 998–1002.

Tallis R (1994) Medical advances and the future of old age. In Marinker M (Ed.) Controversies in Health Care Policies: Challenges to Practice. London: BMJ.

Taylor M B (1997) Compassion: its neglect and importance. British Journal of General Practice 47: 521–5.

Toon P (1994) What is good general practice? Occasional Paper No. 65. London: RCGP.

Tudor Hart J (1988) A New Kind of Doctor. London: Merlin.

Tudor Hart J (1994) Feasible Socialism: the NHS, Past, Present and Future. London: Socialist Health Association.

Vars G F (1991) Integrated curriculum in historical perspective. Educational Leadership (October): 14–15.

Wales E (1978) Behavioural scientist meets the practising physician. Journal of Family Practice 6(4): 839–44.

Wegar K (1992) Sociology in American medical education since the 1960s: the rhetoric of reform. Social Science and Medicine 35(8): 959–65.

Williams G H, Wood P N (1986) Common-sense beliefs about illness: a mediating role for the doctor. Lancet ii: 1435–7.

Wynne-Jones M (1993) General practice: a job for life? British Medical Journal 307: 630.

The way forward

Jane Sims

Recently, there have been various motivators for change in primary care. Whilst economic, political and policy-driven forces are important, one cannot disregard the influence of changes in clinical practice. In addition, the maturation of the general practice, nursing and other health professions should not be discounted. There has been a move towards a greater evaluation of primary care, a growing research and development culture, improved training opportunities and the use of mentors and facilitators to improve the quality of care. Two key processes for gathering information and for monitoring service performance, namely audit and education, have been advanced. Linked to these has been the promulgation of evidence-based practice and healthy professional alliances. More effective use of information technology will play a vital part in extending both clinical, service and educational developments beyond the millennium. To summarize the changes to health care delivery post 1996: the legislation has resulted in a single health strategy for both primary and secondary care. This requires a uniform approach by the health authorities to disease management, purchasing, quality of care, finance and priority-setting across the two sectors. We saw in Chapter 2 that the new organization allows greater liaison with GPs and potentially grants them a greater say in health care policy and services, and forward planning. In Chapter 4, the singular co-ordination of the employment and management of other primary care team members was highlighted as a potential means of benefiting working relationships and easing historical tensions. There is however no panacea: barriers still remain to be overcome, those of financial constraints, obtaining clinical consensus and conflicts between local and national priorities. Whilst UK primary care performed well on Starfield's scoring system, it had a low ranking for health indices and only a moderate one for satisfaction (Starfield, 1992). There is therefore room for improvement.

Not least of the current difficulties facing primary care is the falling recruitment to general practice (Medical Practices Committee, 1996). At a time when the opportunities and challenges for GPs – in service provision, research and education – are increasing, many are asking whether we have enough GPs to do the work (Taylor and Leese, 1997; Wallace et al, 1998). Further steps need to be taken to improve morale and to ensure protected time for non-clinical commitments.

Another quandary is that the move to a primary care-led NHS has not been followed by an adequate shift in resources. Nor are secondary care services less heavily used. The number of people being admitted to hospital has not diminished, although we have no clear evidence why this is. The demand for health care is likely to increase, given the stimulus of demographic, technical and consumer expectations. The examples of counselling in primary care and hospital-at-home schemes demonstrate that, rather than substitution occurring, new services are catering for previously unmet need. The challenge of prioritizing services remains (Cohen, 1994).

The internal market has had its day. Littlejohns (1996) predicted that, given the high costs involved, the lack of competition in certain parts of the country and the unacceptability of 'market losers', there was likely to be a shift towards more collaborative, long-term schemes for purchasing health care. The past decade has seen a reliance on pump-priming funds reacting to problems. We need to view closely the underlying causes of problems and apply longer-term funds to try to address these. In the recent past, the speed with which changes have been adopted has meant a general lack of systematic evaluation. Today's planners need to be mindful of Pettigrew et al's conceptualization of receptive contexts for strategic change (Pettigrew et al, 1992). Harris (1996) has argued that whatever systems evolve, they must be closely monitored and evaluated. He also echoes calls for existing knowledge regarding the effectiveness, efficiency and acceptability of primary care activities and personnel to be properly used to ensure that future ventures are appropriate.

The 1997 White Paper *The New NHS* (Secretary of State for Health, 1997) heralded the end of GP fundholding. In its place, primary care groups are to develop, building on the existing commissioning structures. Primary care groups, consisting of GPs and community nurses, are to work in partnership with health authorities, local authorities and Trusts to ensure quality health care via health improvement programmes. 'Each Primary Care Group will have available their population's share of the available resources for hospital and community health services, prescribing and general practice infrastructure' (Secretary of State for Health, 1997). All GPs will operate within such groupings. All groups will be answerable to health authorities for both financial and clinical matters.

There are four options for the operation of primary care groups, ranging from advising health authorities to taking on legal responsibility for both commissioning care and providing community health services.[1] In the latter case, a new form of Trust is envisaged – a primary care Trust. The aim is to address local needs, within a health improvement programme. Whilst emphasis has been placed on accountability, equity and quality, flexibility exists. There are no artificially capped budgets, for example for emergency services. Primary care groups can decide how best to use their single, unified budget to meet local requirements. Annual contracts are to be replaced by longer-term, 3-year service agreements. These will entail a statutory duty to maintain quality and performance standards. The importance of 'clinical governance' has been emphasized. Primary care groups represent a radical policy initiative and have the potential for far-reaching changes in health care provision.

To promote consistent access to services, standards and guidelines will be extended through the evidence-based national service frameworks. For example, the new national performance framework focuses on accountability to patients. In addition to monitoring efficiency gains, it measures patients' experience of services, fair access to services, improved quality, the outcome of care and improvements in health. As part of this initiative, the NHS is to conduct and publish annual national surveys of patients' and carers' views on NHS services, whilst a revised NHS Charter sets out patients' rights and responsibilities. A National Institute for Clinical Excellence will draw up new guidelines and advice on clinical and cost-effectiveness. The next few years will be exciting for NHS observers watching the development of these initiatives.

The research base in primary care also needs to be strengthened by drawing upon theories from social and organizational sciences as well as clinical science, and from the humanities. Two recent reports have recognized this need and suggest areas for future research (MRC Topic Review Group, 1997; National Working Group on R&D in Primary Care, 1997). They also recommend both support-

[1]It should be noted that specialist services, for example mental health and learning disabilities, will operate outside these Trusts.

ive research training and career structures for primary care professionals.

Given its acknowledged role in cost-effective health care provision, the 'primary care-led NHS' – albeit without this label – will continue into the 21st century. Under the Labour government, collaborative working is to be positively encouraged: indeed, it is viewed as central to the future of the NHS. Service and role integration will be a key feature of the new health action zones. The interface between health and social care is set to expand. Social and health issues will be addressed jointly in broad, community-based developments. We are moving beyond the existing system in which community health services support general practice infrastructure to one that involves local authorities, businesses and the voluntary sector in interagency collaboration.

Hopefully, we will move away from a politically-based to an evidence-based health care agenda, providing proactive, structured care for the promotion of physical and mental health. Patterns of health care provision will necessarily be determined by local circumstances. However, they would benefit from the use of guiding theories rather than being left to develop piecemeal as has often been the case in the past. The Alma-Ata goal of participative and collaborative provision of primary health care remains in sight.

References

Cohen D (1994) Marginal analysis in practice: an alternative to needs assessment for contracting health care. British Medical Journal 309: 781–5.

Harris A (1996) What is a primary care-led policy? In Littlejohns P, Victor C (Eds) Making Sense of a Primary Care-led Service. Oxford: Radcliffe Medical Press.

Littlejohns P (1996) Introduction. In Littlejohns P, Victor C (Eds) Making Sense of a Primary Care-led Service. Oxford: Radcliffe Medical Press.

Medical Practices Committee (1996) Recruitment Survey 1996. London: MPC.

MRC Topic Review Group (1997) Primary Health Care: MRC Topic Review. London: MRC.

National Working Group on R&D in Primary Care (1997) National Working Group on R&D in Primary Care. Final Report. Bristol: NHSE South and West.

Pettigrew A, Ferlie E, McKee L (1992) Shaping Strategic Change. London: Sage Publications.

Secretary of State for Health (1997) The New NHS. London: HMSO.

Starfield B (1992) Primary Care: Concept, Evaluation and Policy. New

York: Oxford University Press.

Taylor DH, Leese B (1997) Recruitment, retention and time commitment change of general practitioners in England and Wales, 1990–1994: a retrospective study. British Medical Journal 314: 1806–12.

Wallace P, Drage S, Jackson N (1998) Linking education, research and service in general practice. British Medical Journal 316: 323.

Appendix: Using the World Wide Web

Once you have access to the World Wide Web, it is possible to perform general searches via any commercial search engine, such as Webcrawler (http://webcrawler.com/). There are also dedicated medical browsers. HealthNet is a computer-based telecommunications system that links health care workers around the world and provides access to the latest medical information (http://www.health-net.org/hnet/hnet.html). OMNI (Organising Medical Networked Information) is a gateway to Internet resources in medicine, biosciences, allied health and health management. It provides a comprehensive coverage of UK resources in this area and access to the best resources worldwide. All resources available through OMNI have been assessed for quality and are reviewed regularly (http://www.omni.ac.uk). Doctors who are members of the British Medical Association have free access to Medline (http://ovid.bma.org.uk). Other sites allowing free access to Medline are listed below. The most useful sources of information on evidence-based practice may be accessed through the Centre for Evidence-based Practice in Oxford (http://cebm.jr2.ox.ac.uk/). It has a number of hypertext links to other sites of interest.

Useful websites

Evidence-based health care websites

- Bandolier – http://www.jr2.ox.ac.uk:80/Bandolier/

This is a monthly journal produced in Oxford for the NHS R&D Directorate. It contains bullet points of evidence-based medicine.

- CASP home page – http://fester.his.path.cam.ac.uk/ phealth/ casphome.htm

CASP is a UK project that aims to promote the delivery of evidence-based health care by helping decision-makers to develop their skills in the critical appraisal of evidence about effectiveness.

- Centre for Evidence-based Child Health – http://www.ich. ucl.ac.uk/ebm/ebm.htm

This is based at the Institute of Child Health in London. The centre runs an educational programme for health professionals that aims to increase the provision of effective and efficient child health care.

- Centre for Evidence-based Dentistry – http://www.bhaoral.demon.co.uk

This is based at the Institute of Health Sciences in Oxford. The aim of the centre is to promote the teaching, learning, practice and evaluation of evidence-based dentistry.

- Clinical Practice Guidelines Program – http://www.amda. ab.ca/general/clinical-practice-guidelines/index.html

This is maintained by the Alberta Medical Association and provides information on the guidelines available for selected topics.

- Cochrane Collaboration – http://hiru.mcmaster.ca/ cochrane/default.htm

The Cochrane Collaboration facilitates the creation, review, maintenance and dissemination of systematic reviews of the effects of health care. The website also contains full-text Cochrane Collaboration manuals.

- AuRACLE – http://panizzi.shef.ac.uk/auracle/aurac.html

Based in the Department of Information Studies at the University of Sheffield, the Automated Retrieval Assistant for Clinically-relevant Evidence project aims to develop a computer-based reference service capable of increasing the range of (evidence-based) information queries that can be handled by machine.

- The NHS Centre for Reviews & Dissemination at York – http://www.york.ac.uk/inst/crd/welcome.htm

The CRD aims to identify and review the results of good quality health research and to disseminate the findings to key decision-makers in the NHS and to consumers of health care services. The reviews cover the effectiveness of care for particular conditions, the effectiveness of health technologies and evidence on efficient methods of organizing and delivering particular types of health care.

- The EBM Project – http://hiru.mcmaster.ca/ebm/ default.htm

Based at McMaster University in Canada, this website features a large inventory of evidence-based resources, including an on-line database, interactive users guides, bibliographies and other useful tools such as the US Prevention Task Force Guides to Clinical Preventive Services.

Electronic journal clubs

- ACP Journal Club – http://hiru.mcmaster.ca/acpjc/ default.htm

ACP aims to select articles from the biomedical literature that report studies and reviews warranting immediate attention by physicians attempting to keep pace with important advances in internal medicine. These articles are summarized in 'value-added' abstracts and commented on by clinical experts.

- Journal Club on the WEB – http://www.webcom.com/ mjljweb/jrnlclb/about.html

This is an interactive medical journal club run by Michael Jacobson. Two or three times a month, he summarizes and comments on an article from the recent medical literature. The articles are primarily in the field of adult internal medicine and mainly from the *New England Journal of Medicine*, *Annals of Internal Medicine*, *Journal of the American Medical Association* and the *Lancet*.

- The Journal of Family Practice Journal Club – http://jfp.msu.edu/

The Journal Club reviews seven to ten articles from the primary care literature each month as part of POEMs (Patient-Oriented Evidence that Matters).

Free access to Medline

- Avicenna – http://www.avicenna.com/

- BioMedNet's Evaluated Medline – http://biomednet.com/db/medline

- CME-CE.COM – http://www.cme-ce.com/medline/

- Healthworks MEDLINEPlus – http://www.healthworks.co.uk/hw/medline/medline.html

- Medscape – http://www.medscape.com/

Index